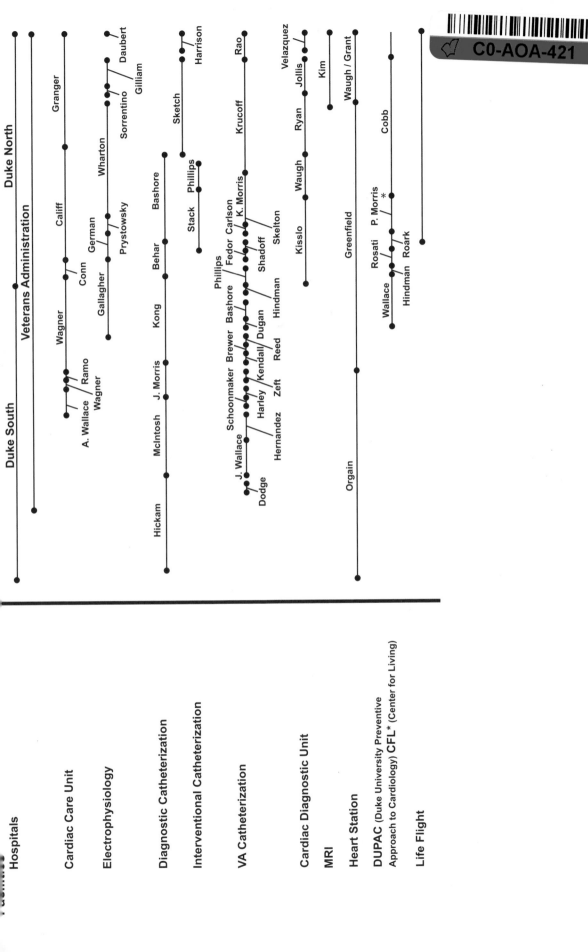

Duke Cardiology Fellows Training Program

Duke Cardiology Fellows Training Program

Sixty-three Years of Excellence

To Harry

Best Wishes
Joe Greenfield

Joseph C. Greenfield, Jr., MD

CAROLINA ACADEMIC PRESS
Durham, North Carolina

Library of Congress Cataloging-in-Publication Data

Greenfield, Joseph C.
  Duke cardiology fellows training program : sixty-three years of excellence / Joseph C.
Greenfield Jr.
    p. ; cm.
  ISBN 978-1-59460-969-5 (alk. paper)
  1. Duke University. Medical Center. Cardiology Fellows Training Program. 2. Cardi-
ology--History. 3. Medical colleges--North Carolina--History. I. Title.
  [DNLM: 1. Duke Cardiology Fellows Training Program. 2. Cardiology--education--
North Carolina. 3. Cardiology--history--North Carolina. 4. Fellowships and Scholar-
ships--history--North Carolina. 5. History, 20th Century--North Carolina. 6. His-
tory, 21st Century--North Carolina. 7. Schools, Medical--history--North Carolina.
WG 11 AN8]

  R747.D817G74 2011
  610.71'1756563--dc22

                        2010053670

Carolina Academic Press
700 Kent Street
Durham, NC 27701
Telephone (919) 489-7486
Fax (919) 493-5668
www.cap-press.com

It is with a great deal of appreciation that this book is dedicated to the Cardiology Fellows. For over six decades, their unfailing commitment has made the Duke Cardiology Division without peer.

CONTENTS

PREFACE

As a general rule, the purpose of a Preface is to provide the reader with the author's justification or defense, as the case may be, of what has been written. If adequate, it should entice the reader to delve further into the body of the book. I hope that the Preface accomplishes this goal.

For more than 60 years, graduates of the Cardiology Fellows Training Program at Duke University Medical Center have made a major positive impact on the treatment of patients with cardiovascular disease. These physicians have been at the forefront of developing strategies for improving health care, carrying out both clinical and basic research, delivering outstanding patient care, and training future cardiologists.

What are the strategies which this or, in fact, any Training Program must augment in order to assure the development of outstanding cardiologists? The primary precepts are really quite simple. 1) Recruit the highest quality, dedicated physicians as trainees and 2) provide a milieu where every aspect of their training is designed to inculcate the cognitive and philosophical components of an outstanding physician. Thus, it is mandatory that in every aspect of training, be it patient care or research, only the highest quality approaches are acceptable. The achievement of these goals is in constant need of reaffirmation by all those involved with the Training Program. Frankly, without constant surveillance, any Training Program will slip into mediocrity. I believe that our Cardiology Training Program has met these criteria at the highest level.

The primary purpose of this book is not only to document these achievements, but also to examine the nature of the Training Program and to whatever extent possible, define the factors which have led to the outstanding results.

This programmatic description encompasses the period from 1946 through 2009. The material in this manuscript has been extensively revised and enlarged since the original publication: *Duke Cardiology Fellows Training Program, Origin to the Present*, published in 2004.

Throughout the manuscript, the designation "fellow" denotes a physician either during or after finishing their fellowship. In order to be included, a fellow must have been enrolled in the Training Program for at least one year.

In presenting the large body of material, Chapters II–VII deal with specific time periods. Each of these chapters presents both a narrative of the programmatic development as well as a Table listing the names of the fellows, the types of training and future careers. (A detailed explanation of the content of these Tables is given at the end of Chapter II.) The remaining chapters deal with specific aspects of the Training Program.

The Appendix documents the sources of the data. A "Rogues' Gallery" contains pictures obtained usually in a non-academic setting of a number of the fellows and faculty.

In order to provide a visual overview, significant milestones in the development of the Cardiology Division and the Cardiology Fellows Training Program are illustrated by the Frontispiece.

Acknowledgments

There are a number of people who have been extraordinarily helpful in developing this material.

Bettie Houston has been responsible primarily for locating the graduates and obtaining pertinent material from them. This was a monumental effort. In addition, she meticulously prepared multiple drafts of the data tables and the manuscript. As always, she carried out the work gracefully and with good humor.

Judith Rembert has been instrumental in acquiring, sifting through, organizing and editing the voluminous material. It is difficult to succinctly characterize her multiple contributions: probably best expressed as quality control.

Drs. Galen Wagner, Tom Bashore and Chris O'Connor have been essential resources and have made numerous helpful observations and suggestions.

Dr. Bob Waugh functioned as the primary photographer.

Financial support was obtained from the Institute for Medical Research at the Durham Veterans Affairs Medical Center, the Division of Cardiology and the Heart Center, Duke University Medical Center, and the Duke Endowment due to Dr. William G. Anlyan.

A number of the Cardiology faculty and fellows have allowed me to "pick their brains" regarding their perspectives of the Fellowship Training Program.

Finally, it would be amiss not to recognize the efforts of my fellow Chiefs of Cardiology: Drs. Henry McIntosh, Andy Wallace, Gary Stiles, Pascal Goldschmidt, Pam Douglas and Howard Rockman along with the Training Program Directors—Drs. Galen Wagner, Ed Pritchett, Gary Stiles, Tom Bashore and Andrew Wang. Their leadership over the years has shaped and nurtured the Training Program.

Dr. Eugene A. Stead, Jr. (1908–2005) made of number of unique contributions which fostered the development of the Training Program.

Special recognition is given to Dr. Edward S. Orgain (1906–1995), who not only initiated the Training Program, but also served as an outstanding role model for nearly 40 years.

Duke Cardiology Fellows Training Program

CHAPTER I

ORIGIN

The mission to develop subspecialty training in cardiology was surprisingly quite late in being implemented at Duke University Medical Center (DUMC). Dr. Christopher Johnston, a cardiologist trained at Johns Hopkins University, was recruited by Dean Wilburt C. Davison in 1930 to be a member of the original Department of Medicine faculty.[1] Dr. Edward S. Orgain, a product of the Cardiovascular Training Program at Massachusetts General Hospital, led by Dr. Paul Dudley White, joined the staff in 1934. After Dr. Johnston resigned in 1946, Dr. Orgain was the sole cardiologist at Duke Medical Center.[2]

During his tenure, Dr. Orgain had developed a very large and high quality cardiology practice and was quite active in teaching both medical students and house staff. In addition, he published a number of manuscripts dealing with cardiovascular diseases, especially bacterial endocarditis. Thus, all the necessary components for the establishment of a training program in cardiology seemed to have been in place by the late 1930s.

Undoubtedly, the medical manpower needs of World War II, in large measure, prevented the widespread development of training programs in the medical subspecialties. In general, physicians, following minimal house staff training, became involved immediately in the war effort so that extensive post-graduate education was impossible. However, in the aftermath of World War II, the manpower situation changed dramatically. A number of physicians sought additional specific training in the medical subspecialties—cardiology among them. To meet this need, in July of 1946, Dr. Orgain appointed Drs. Lee Messer and Charles Donegan as cardiology fellows.

The Duke Cardiology Fellows Training Program was formally launched.

CHAPTER II

1946–59

The fledgling Cardiology Training Program received a significant boost when Dr. Eugene A. Stead, a nationally known cardiovascular physiologist and cardiologist, arrived at Duke in 1947 as the Chairman of the Department of Medicine. Dr. Stead felt strongly that fostering post-graduate education should be a primary function for the Department. An "unsolicited" training grant from the National Heart Institute (NHI) was awarded to Dr. Stead. He designated a yearly stipend to support a trainee available to Dr. Orgain. This grant enabled at least one fellow to be fully funded and gave significant financial stability to the Program (Chapter X).

Although there were occasional exceptions, at least during the first decade, the Training Program in Cardiology directed by Dr. Orgain required a two-year commitment. In general, two fellows were accepted each year, resulting in a steady state group of four. The Program was centered around the care of patients with cardiovascular disease. Dr. Orgain served as the primary mentor. Patient care and teaching rounds on the inpatient services were held each morning with Dr. Orgain. A cardiology on-call service was developed and the responsibilities divided among the fellows. Along with the house staff, the fellows were responsible for evaluating all patients admitted to both Dr. Orgain's private service and those seen in consultation.[1]

It should be remembered that, at this time, there was no Cardiac Care Unit. The treatment of patients with acute myocardial infarction involved a prolonged (four to six weeks) period of essentially strict bed rest. Many of the sequela following acute myocardial infarction were related specifically to this therapy: e.g., venous thrombosis, shoulder-hand syndrome and debilitating deconditioning. The daily care of these patients and maintaining an appropriate liaison with their families was a prime responsibility of the fellows. The trainees also evaluated patients in the Cardiology Clinics, both private and public.

The fellows were responsible for interpreting all the electrocardiograms recorded at Duke Hospital. They held a teaching session for house staff and students each afternoon at 5:00 p.m. The problem electrocardiograms were reviewed with Dr. Orgain the next day at noon. ECG recordings were carried out with a string galvanometer and processed by an antiquated photographic technique. Since the recordings had to be developed, the electrocardiogram could not be viewed immediately. (Direct-writing electrocardiographic instruments were not in general use at Duke Hospital until the mid 1960s).

The fellows were responsible for performing a number of diagnostic and therapeutic procedures.[1] Electrocardiographic measurement of exercise-induced myocardial ischemia required "hands on" participation by the fellows. A treadmill was unavailable. The exercise protocol, a variant of the Master "two-step" test, was carried out with the patient and the fellow walking up and down a flight of steps located near the Heart

Station. The exercise was continued until the patient became fatigued, dyspneic or had chest pain. (This process kept the fellows in reasonably good physical condition.) Cardioversion of atrial fibrillation or flutter with oral quinidine was supervised by the fellows. Cardiac rhythms were diagnosed by esophageal electrocardiograms obtained by the fellows. Cardiac evaluation of patients usually included a chest fluoroscopy and barium swallow carried out by the fellows in conjunction with Dr. Orgain.

The Cardiac Catheterization Laboratory was developed and supervised by Dr. John Hickam, a cardiopulmonary physiologist who had arrived with Dr. Stead. The primary function of this laboratory was research, but selected clinical patients were evaluated. The fellows had the option of training in right heart cardiac catheterization techniques, but it was not required. Shortly after Dr. Hickam left in 1958, Dr. Henry McIntosh became the Director of the Cardiac Catheterization Laboratory.

There were several outside clinical activities available for the fellows, including functioning as a consulting cardiologist at the Fayetteville Veterans Administration (VA) Hospital. These were eagerly sought because they provided additional salary funds. The fellow stipend initially was $2400/year and did not increase significantly for nearly a ten-year period.

The Program did not have specific didactic course work or lectures. The fellows did attend Medical Grand Rounds and were required to prepare didactic lectures for house staff and medical students. In addition, they participated in the teaching of physical diagnosis to the students.

The Cardiothoracic Surgery Service headed by Dr. Will Sealy was quite active. He developed techniques to repair congenital and rheumatic valvular abnormalities which could be approached without the necessity of cardiopulmonary bypass. Under the direction of Dr. Ivan Brown, open heart surgery became a reality at Duke in 1956. Initially, this procedure was utilized primarily to repair atrial septal defects. Since there was a large backlog of patients, cardiology fellows spent a considerable period of time evaluating these patients both pre and post operatively.

Dr. Orgain always had a keen interest in clinical descriptions of patients with cardiovascular disease; during his fellowship with Dr. White, published several papers. One of the primary clinical research interests of Dr. Orgain was the treatment of hypertension. Dr. Walter Kempner, of Rice Diet fame, had a large cadre of patients receiving dietary treatment for hypertension. Dr. Orgain became interested in the use of antihypertensive drugs (hexamethonium, reserpine and apresoline) and to some extent two "competing programs" to treat hypertension resulted. One of the early descriptions of the lupus-like syndrome associated with apresoline was published by Dr. Orgain and his fellows. In addition, he carried out a number of studies on long-acting nitrates to treat angina. The fellows were always encouraged to participate in these studies and the majority availed themselves of the opportunity. Almost without exception, the fellows published manuscripts on a variety of topics relating to the cardiovascular system during their fellowship.

Although the Program developed by Dr. Orgain was the primary locus for clinical training in cardiology, other opportunities were developed to promote cardiovascular research and clinical training. The Durham VA Hospital (DVAH) had been formally opened in 1953 and Dr. James V. Warren, a well-known cardiovascular physiologist and a colleague of Dr. Stead's at Emory University, had been recruited to be Chief of Medicine. Dr. Warren recruited Dr. Hal Dodge who had a specific research interest in ventricular function as assessed by ventricular volume measurements. In addition as noted, Dr. Hickam had an active research program in cardiopulmonary physiology.

Several fellows were recruited to carry out hemodynamic research under the tutelage of Drs. Stead, Warren, Hickam: e.g., Drs. Arnie Weissler, Jim Leonard, Jack Wallace, and Harvey Estes became trainees in this environment. Their primary function was cardiovascular research. However, they did participate in the teaching program at both the DUMC inpatient and outpatient services and at the DVAH but had no assigned subspecialty training in cardiology. Although an extraordinarily talented group, one wonders on what basis was this level of clinical experience in cardiology considered to be acceptable for admission to the subspecialty board examination in Cardiovascular Disease? When asked this question, Dr. Stead responded, "I was a good letter writer".

Dr. Warren left to become Chairman of Medicine at the University of Texas at Galveston in 1956 and Dr. Hickam left to be Chairman of Medicine at Indiana University in 1958.

In 1956, Dr. Estes became a senior staff cardiologist with a primary function in the Private Diagnostic Clinic. His clinical service was separate from Dr. Orgain's. The trainees were involved with Dr. Estes only to the extent that since he was a highly experienced electrocardiographer, he taught electrocardiography to the fellows, house staff and students. In July 1959, Dr. Estes became Chief of Medicine at the DVAH. Dr. Bill Floyd, who had been a fellow for two years with Dr. Orgain, became a faculty member. The clinical practice of Drs. Orgain and Floyd became known as the Cardiovascular Disease Service. Dr. Bob Whalen joined this service shortly thereafter.

Dr. McIntosh, who had been Chief Resident at the DVAH in 1954, initially became involved with the development of the renal dialysis program. However, as noted, Dr. McIntosh became the Director of the Cardiac Catheterization Laboratory following Dr. Hickam's departure. In 1958, this function moved to new quarters below a small store, affectionately known as the "Dope Shop", near Dean Davison's office. Shortly thereafter, Dr. McIntosh initiated a formal two-year Training Program in both clinical cardiology and cardiovascular research, using the catheterization laboratory as the primary locus for these activities. Drs. Tommy Thompson and Bill Gleason were the initial trainees; thereafter two fellows per year were accepted.

The majority of the procedures were right ventricular catheterization. (Angiography was not available for several years.) Left ventricular catheterization, rarely employed, was approached by retrograde aortic catheterization. In conjunction with Dr Sealy, measurement of left atrial pressure was carried out through a bronchoscope.

An additional opportunity for training in cardiovascular disease at this time should be noted. All physicians were subject to the "doctor draft" and as such were deferred through their house staff training by the Berry Plan. (They had a two-year commitment to the armed services at the end of their training.) In many cases, service in the military involved significant subspecialty training along with the clinical duties. Obviously, the training opportunities depended on a specific assignment. Trying to estimate the amount of cardiology training during the military service is essentially impossible. Suffice to say, the training careers of the majority of the fellows entering the Program up to the mid-1970s were significantly augmented by military service.

A unique opportunity was provided at the Clinical Center of the National Institutes of Health which had opened its doors for patients in 1955. Physicians were needed to take care of the patients hospitalized for clinical research. Physicians selected to this program were in the Public Health Service and their commitments to the "doctor draft" thus were fulfilled. Dr. Andy Wallace (1961–1963) and I (1959–62) participated in this program at the National Heart Institute (NHI). I returned to be a Clinical Investigator at the DVAH and Andy to be Chief Resident in Medicine at Duke Hospital.

Table 1 Cardiology Fellows: 1946–59

Name	Institution Internship/Residency	Fellowship Dates	Clinical Category	Research	Initial Career	Subsequent Career
Bacos, James M.	Duke Medical Center	1956–57 1958–59	G	C	A	P
Broome, Robert A.	Jefferson-Hillman, Birmingham Duke Medical Center	1948–50	G		P	P, Dec
Bryant, Gerald N.	Duke Medical Center	1957–59	G	C	P	P, Ret
Donegan, Charles K.	Duke Medical Center	1946–48	G		P	P, Dec
Donnelly, George L. (Laurie)	New South Wales, Australia	1955–57*	G		P	P, Dec
Eagan, Sr., John T.	Duke Medical Center	1958–60	G		P	P
Estes, Jr., E. Harvey	Emory—Grady Duke Medical Center	1952–53	G	C	A	A, Ret
Floyd, Walter L. (Bill)	Johns Hopkins Grace, New Haven Hosp. Duke Medical Center	1957–59	G		A	A, Ret
Gibbons, James E.	Ottawa Civic Hosp., Ottawa, Canada Royal Victoria Hosp., Montreal, Canada	1954–56*	G–PED		A	A, Dec
Gleason, William L.	Duke Medical Center—CR Cincinnati General Hosp.	1957–59*	G–IV	C	P	P, Ret
Greenfield, Jr., Joseph C.	Duke Medical Center	1959–62*	G	B	A	A
Hair, Jr., Thomas E.	Parkland—UTSW Duke Medical Center U. North Carolina	1959–61	G		P	P, Dec

Name	Institution Internship/Residency	Fellowship Dates	Clinical Category	Research	Initial Career	Subsequent Career
Izlar, H. LeRoy (Roy)	Vanderbilt; Bowman Gray; Duke Medical Center	1954–55	G		P	P, Dec
Leonard, James J.	Georgetown	1956–57*	G	C	A	A, Ret, Dec
Maha, George E.	Mount Carmel Mercy Hosp., Detroit; St. Louis University/Cochrane VA Hosp.	1956–58	G		P	OMI, Ret
McIntosh, Henry D.	Duke Medical Center—CR; Lawson General Hosp., Atlanta	1952–54	G–IV	C	A	A, P, Ret, Dec
Messer, Addison L. (Lee)	Bellevue Hosp., NYC; Mass. General Hosp.	1946–48*	G		P	P, Dec
Miller, D. Edmond (Ed)	Duke Medical Center	1958–59, 61	G		P	P, Ret
Muller, John C.	Duke Medical Center	1952–54	G		P	P, Dec
Munroe, Colin A.	Duke Medical Center	1957	G		P	P, Dec
Pryor, William W. (Putt)	Duke Medical Center	1952–56	G	C	P	P, Ret
Rast, Jr., Charles L.	Duke Medical Center; Johns Hopkins	1952–54	G		P	P, Ret
Roehll, Jr., Walter H.	Cincinnati General Hosp.—CR	1959–60	G	C	P	P
Shapiro, O. William (Bill)	Duke Medical Center; Mount Sinai, NYC	1956–57*	G	C	A	A, Dec
Sieber, Homer A.	U. Virginia, Charlottesville	1951–53	G		P	P, Dec
Sleeper, Julian C.	Vanderbilt; Duke Medical Center	1959–62	G		P	P, Ret
Thompson, Howard K. (Tommy)	Bellevue Hosp., NYC; Duke Medical Center—CR	1958–60*	G–IV	C	A	A, P, Ret, Dec

Name	Institution Internship/Residency	Fellowship Dates	Clinical Category	Research	Initial Career	Subsequent Career
Voyles, Carl M.	Johns Hopkins Duke Medical Center	1950–52	G		P	OM, P, Ret, P
Wallace, John M. (Jack)	Duke Medical Center New York Hosp., NYC St. Louis City Hosp.—CR	1955–58	G	B	A	A, Ret
Weissler, Arnold M.	Maimonides Hosp., Brooklyn	1955–57	G	C	A	A, Ret

Explanation for Data Tables

Fellows

The Tables following Chapters II–VII encompass a specific time period (usually ten years). Fellows are listed in a table based on the date of their <u>entry</u> into the Program.

<u>Name</u>: Names on a given table appear in alphabetical order. The familiar name, if not obvious from the given name, is listed in parenthesis. A closed circle following a name indicates that data regarding the individual has not been obtained for the preceding five years.

<u>Institution</u>: The institution(s) is listed where the individual trained in Internal Medicine. (CR) indicates Chief Residency.

<u>Fellowship</u> <u>Dates</u>: Since the duration of most fellowships is from July – June, both years are given. An asterisk indicates that the fellow had additional cardiology training, either research or clinical, at another institution.

<u>Clinical</u> <u>Category</u>: General [without intensive training in procedures], (G). Electrophysiology, (EP). Interventional [intensive cardiac catheterization without angioplasty], (IV). Interventional [including angioplasty], (IC). Noninvasive [echocardiography, and/or nuclear imaging, and/or magnetic resonance imaging], (NIV). Rehabilitation, (REH). Combined both adult and pediatric, (PED). Other, transfer to a different medical specialty, (O).

<u>Research</u>: As a general rule, most fellows carried out clinical research during their fellowship. An entry in this column is reserved for those spending at least six months dedicated time in research. Clinical (C) implies that the research is descriptive in nature and generally is carried out in patients. Basic (B) is defined as research that is mechanistic in nature and is carried out either in patients, animals, or a "bench" laboratory.

<u>Initial</u> <u>Career</u>: The one-year period following completion of the fellowship is designated as the initial career. The specific job designations are as follows: Academic (A) implies an academic position with a specific duty. Academic also will be designated if the individual has an academic appointment, but is located in a hospital which is affiliated with an academic institution and carries out significant teaching or research activities. A full-time position at the National Institutes of Health, Food and Drug Administration, or at an institution having a training program in cardiology, e.g., the Scripps Clinic, is considered academic. (An additional year taken as an Associate, which was a continuation of the fellowship, is not listed as an initial career.) Practice (P) denotes engaged in the practice of cardiology in a non-academic setting. The individual may have a clinical or consulting academic appointment. Additional career designations include: full-time military (OM), medical industry such as pharmaceutical or medical device (OMI), another medical specialty such as surgery, a non-medical field such as legal, or pursuing another academic degree (O).

<u>Subsequent</u> <u>Career</u>: The subsequent career begins at the end of the first post-fellowship year. Designations are the same as in the previous category. More than one entry denotes significant changes within this category. The last entry indicates the

current position or the position held when the individual retired (Ret) or died (Dec). The designation (Ret) indicates that the individual is not engaged in either significant part-time practice or academic work. A two to three year period in military service in order to fulfill the "doctor draft" requirements is not designated as a specific category.

CHAPTER III

1960–69

By 1960, Dr. Stead had stopped mentoring individual fellows and both Drs. Hickam and Warren had left the institution. As a result, only two cardiology training opportunities remained: 1) the Cardiovascular Disease Service directed by Dr. Orgain and 2) the Cardiac Catheterization Laboratory directed by Dr. McIntosh. The training format for the former remained essentially as described previously. Although there were exceptions, the fellows during the initial years of this decade worked in one or the other Program without significant crossover.

Trainees in the Cardiac Catheterization Laboratory were expected to become proficient in both current and newly developing catheterization techniques: e.g., transeptal catheterization and somewhat later, coronary arteriography. The majority of the patients had either valvular or congenital heart disease. (Coronary artery bypass surgery did not begin at DUMC until 1968.) The fellows attended outpatient cardiology clinics, but did not have specific inpatient responsibilities.

The primary teaching function was carried out in a daily afternoon conference. All patients scheduled for cardiac catheterization procedures the following day were examined along with the ancillary data (electrocardiogram, phonocardiogram, etc.). A differential diagnosis was developed and the necessary invasive procedures for the next day were determined. In addition, the results of the day's studies were compared to the pre-catheterization assessments. This conference was considered by many of the attendees as the "best teaching experience" they ever had. In addition, attendance was mandatory at a weekly conference held in conjunction with the thoracic surgeons and the pediatric cardiologists in which patients were evaluated for cardiac surgery.

The main thrust of the clinical research centered on the development of cine angiographic techniques to measure ventricular volumes. These data formed the basis of a number of studies of cardiac function; e.g., hypertrophic subaortic stenosis.

The Catheterization Laboratory was used to carry out a number of studies of cardiac function in a variety of animals; e.g., dogs, pigs, alligators and turkeys—to name a few. Obviously, laboratory schedules had to be developed so that the same facilities could be used for both human and animal studies. A number of interesting situations occurred with this format—none detrimental to either patient care or animal husbandry.

The alligators did present somewhat of a problem—they could not be cajoled to lie still during the procedure. Prior to the study, they were cooled in the laboratory refrigerator. The trick was to have the alligator torpid enough to be still but not so cold that the heart would beat less than once per minute. Sometimes it worked, sometimes it didn't. When it didn't, a lively alligator crawling around the laboratory had to be subdued.

Dr. Tommy Thompson relates an interesting episode from one of the "turkey studies". This experiment, not a survival study, took place near Thanksgiving. The turkey, a quite handsome bird, weighed nearly 20 pounds. Someone came up with a particularly bright idea: have the bird participate in the annual Thanksgiving feast. In due course, the animal was cooked and served to the laboratory staff. Everything seemed fine until the first bite. Unfortunately, the turkey had been anesthetized with ether. The tissues permeated with this substance, to say the least, were not appetizing. (Luckily the main dish did not explode during cooking.) At any rate, the Thanksgiving feast proceeded—sans turkey.

By mid decade, the Hyperbaric Program expanded into a separate building constructed to house several "diving" facilities. Several of the fellows participated in research studies in hyperbaric medicine.

Rapidly developing technology resulted in multiple and dramatic changes in the practice of cardiology. Electrical techniques for both permanent and temporary cardiac pacing became available. Placement of temporary intra-cardiac pacing electrodes was carried out in the Cardiac Catheterization Laboratory. Implantation of permanent pacemakers required the leads to be sewed directly to the surface of the heart and was under the purview of the Thoracic Surgery Service.

Another innovative advance included the use of electrical shock for the treatment of atrial fibrillation and ventricular tachycardia and fibrillation. The first such unit at Duke was housed in a very large, immobile and heavy rack containing a defibrillator and a small ECG monitoring scope. For reasons now lost in the mists of time, the instrument was dubbed "Clyde". One of Clyde's initial functions was described by Dr. Jim Morris.

On the day that Jim began his Chief Residency at Duke, he and his wife were involved in an altercation with the coal delivery train while driving to work. Their car and both of them came off decidedly second best. Although apparently not seriously injured, Mary Ann suffered a blow to her chest. During the subsequent evaluation, she was found to have multiple premature ventricular contractions. Hence, the question arose as to whether or not she had a significant contusion of the heart. She was admitted to DUMC for observation. Clyde was placed in her room, disassembled so that the monitor could be watched from outside her hospital door. Drs. McIntosh, Stead and several other cardiologists took turns for 48 hours watching her electrocardiogram on the monitor. No untoward events occurred. Cardiac monitoring at Duke had become a reality!

Following his Chief Residency, Dr. Andy Wallace wanted to do research in basic electrophysiology. Laboratory space was essentially non-existent. In a stroke of good fortune, Dr. Will Sealy welcomed Andy's research program into his laboratory facilities. Several fellows were attracted to work in this program and received their cardiology training primarily in this venue. One of the major research interests was the study of atrial activation. These studies resulted in the development of a successful surgical approach to the ablation of bypass tracks in Wolff-Parkinson-White syndrome (WPW). The sequence of events leading up to the development of this procedure is described by Dr. Fred Cobb, a fellow at that time.

"Each Saturday morning a research conference was held to review the status of research and to review pertinent articles from the literature. Based on two articles, the treatment of WPW was a topic of discussion at one of these meetings. In one report, the tachycardia in a group of patients had been terminated by appropriately positioned atrial stimulation via a pacing wire in the atrium. The second article documented an unsuccessful attempt to surgically interrupt a bypass track in a patient with WPW who was undergoing repair of an atrial septal defect. Shortly after this research conference (February 1968), Mr. Norman Salter, a 32 year old fisherman from the North Carolina outerbanks, was admitted to the Cardiac Care Unit. He had a history of frequent episodes of tachycardia and the recent onset of signs and symptoms suggesting congestive heart failure. During this admission, he had intermittent episodes of tachycardia (150–180 b.p.m.) lasting from minutes to several hours. When the patient was in sinus rhythm, the electrocardiogram demonstrated Type B WPW conduction. The arrhythmia was unaffected by administration of digitalis, quinidine, diphenylhydantoin or propranolol. An isopotential body surface map, recorded by Dr. Jack Boineau, suggested that anomalous ventricular excitation occurred at the lateral aspect of the right atrioventricular groove. The case was discussed with Dr. Sealy; he decided to attempt to surgically interrupt the bypass track. At the time of surgery, epicardial mapping was performed and the earliest area of ventricular activation identified. An incision in this area abolished the early activation as well as the electrocardiographic features of WPW. Postoperatively, the tachycardia ceased and the symptoms of congestive heart failure rapidly subsided. Mr. Salter returned to work as a fisherman. A 20 year follow-up revealed no evidence of recurrence of the arrhythmia or heart failure."

Following the unequivocal success of this procedure, a number of patients were referred for similar treatment. In fact, for a number of years at Duke, the correction of WPW became the highest volume surgical procedure for congenital heart disease. The widespread notoriety was an important factor in attracting outstanding fellows to the Cardiology Training Program.

Upon returning from the NHI, I began a series of studies to define the instantaneous relationships between aortic blood pressure and flow in patients with a wide variety of cardiac diseases. A newly refurbished Cardiac Catheterization Laboratory at the DVAH was utilized for these procedures. Fellows began to participate in these research studies, and at the same time, learned cardiac catheterization techniques. Beginning with Dr. Ralph Hernandez, a training path was developed in which selected fellows received in-depth training in catheterization techniques. Following this training, they became Chief of the DVAH Catheterization Laboratory for the next one to three years. This very successful format continued for approximately the next 25 years (see Frontispiece). The facilities at the DVAH began to be used by other fellows to train in all aspects of cardiology. For the subsequent decade, a number of fellows received the bulk of their training at the DVAH.

The rapid progression of technology to treat patients with acute myocardial infarction (electrical pacing for rhythm control, defibrillation and precise hemodynamic monitoring) stimulated the development of dedicated Cardiac Care Units (CCU) in many academic centers. Dr. Wallace took the leadership role in organizing the CCU. A wing of Drake Ward was refurbished and in December 1965, the Duke CCU became a reality.

Unfortunately, this location for the CCU limited access from the medical wards in the front of the hospital (Drake and Minot) to those in the back (Osler and Long). Closing this corridor was not well received by a number of the medical staff physicians. In fact, in spite of the "rules" to the contrary, the CCU continued to be used as a walkway. Although generally detrimental to maintaining a quiet environment, one notably positive incident occurred. While traipsing through the CCU, Dr. Hal Silberman, a member of the Hematology-Oncology Division, was passing by the room occupied by Dr. J. Lamar Callaway (Chief of Dermatology). Dr. Callaway had just been admitted with an acute inferior myocardial infarction. Hal happened to glance at the monitor at the instant ventricular fibrillation occurred. He acted immediately, grabbed the paddles and successfully resuscitated the patient. (As a result, Dr. Callaway lived a productive life for over 30 years.) At least in this case, "All's Well That Ends Well". Although it took awhile, the excess traffic through the CCU did finally cease.

By the summer of 1966, two fellows, Drs. Rick Schaal and Doug Zipes, who had been studying basic electrophysiology, became involved in the care of these patients — an additional training opportunity became a reality. This research and training effort was facilitated by an award in 1968 from the NHI to specifically study patients with acute myocardial infarction (MIRU – Myocardial Infarction Research Unit). The funds from this award provided salary support for both fellows and senior staff cardiologists along with a sophisticated computer to be used for online hemodynamic monitoring. Thus, the majority of the patients admitted to the CCU were involved in a series of clinical investigations.

One of the interesting outgrowths from the MIRU involved the availability of a high-speed (for that time) computer. The purpose for this instrument was based on the experience of Dr. John Kirklin, Chief of Surgery at Alabama, who had found that computers could be employed to monitor cardiac patients following open heart surgery. The MIRU Units were charged with testing how valuable this approach might be in the care of patients with acute myocardial infarction. A number of algorithms for hemodynamic monitoring were developed. However, it became rather obvious over the next two years that a well-trained CCU nurse could not be supplanted by a computer: Hence, the excitement involved in extensive computer-based hemodynamic monitoring began to wane. Cardiology had a problem: what to do with a very expensive computer with considerable capability and no definite plans for its use?

As he had done many times in the past, Dr. Stead's fertile imagination came to the rescue. For several years Dr. Stead had espoused the concept of a computer-based "Textbook of Medicine". The idea was based on the notion that doctors have a limited memory. Clinical decisions are made on the outcome of the last few patients treated. Since the computer would not have a memory lapse, information placed in the computer could be made available for doctors to immediately query large series of patient outcomes. Hence, the practice of medicine would be based on a firm foundation.

When Frank Starmer, PhD who directed the MIRU Computer Facility, initiated this project, the Cardiology Databank was born. Dr. Galen Wagner, who had replaced Andy Wallace in 1968 as the CCU Director, worked with Frank to collect and codify clinical data on patients with acute myocardial infarction. Galen developed a mechanism for the collection of follow-up information. Soon it became evident that this approach provided an excellent opportunity to carry out clinical research. The Duke Databank became established as an important venue for training fellows in clinical investigation.

As part of the MIRU project, an area was provided on the CCU to house equipment, etc. This was rapidly transformed into a procedure area for hemodynamic monitoring. Also, it began to be used for the insertion of pacing electrodes for temporary cardiac pacing. This facility became the "home" for the Clinical Electrophysiology Laboratory.

In 1967, Dr. Stead retired as Chairman of the Department of Medicine and was followed by Dr. James B. Wyngaarden. Dr. Wyngaarden made a number of appointments which strengthened the divisional structure of the Department. Although Dr. Orgain retained the title of Chief of the Cardiovascular Disease Service, Dr. Henry McIntosh became the first Chief of the Cardiology Division in January 1968.

Dr. Jim Morris replaced Dr. McIntosh as Chief of the Catheterization Laboratory. New and expanded laboratory facilities were occupied. Since it was not feasible to continue to carry out animal research in the new facilities, an animal research laboratory was constructed at the Animal Farm on Duke Homestead Road. Thus ended the mixing of patient and animal studies in the same laboratory.

Dr. Bob Whalen, who had a brief unrewarding experience as Medical Director of Duke Hospital, elected to rejoin Drs. Floyd and Orgain in the Cardiovascular Disease Service.

Dr. McIntosh, as always, took his new responsibilities very seriously and involved a number of the members of the Division in helping to solve problems. Although not specifically related to training, the following is illustrative.

In order to deal with the plans for divisional growth, Dr. McIntosh had a penchant for early morning meetings. At least once a week, he met with the physicians from the various components of Cardiology at 7:00 a.m. for "Operation Needle". What seemed to be of paramount importance, at least to me, was refurbishing Minot Ward. When built, Duke Hospital did not provide private bathrooms for each room—the ward contained only a communal bathroom. While this approach seemed reasonable for the 1930s and 40s, by the current decade it was clearly an antiquated situation and made it difficult to attract patients. Thus, plans had to be devised to provide toilet facilities for each of the patient rooms. Since these rooms were small, a separate walled-off enclosure for a bathroom was impossible. Week after week, from 7:00 – 8:00 a.m., we poured over various drawings; no viable solution seemed feasible. Finally, after a somewhat long and unrewarding early morning discussion, I came up with a somewhat radical idea. "Why not hang them from the ceiling upside down?" Dr. McIntosh took considerable umbrage to my suggestion and went on a major pout. I was not invited back. For me, the early morning meetings came to an end. To rephrase a famous quote, "Frankly, I didn't give a damn".

In spite of the propensity for excessive meetings, all aspects of the Division flourished dramatically under Dr. McIntosh's tutelage. Training continued to be of paramount importance. Dr. McIntosh immediately set about to define and unify the structure of the Fellowship Program.

In 1968, the first schedule for fellow appointments and activities was developed. It contains 19 names and five different training areas. Although the opportunity was available for the fellows to move from one training area to another, even by the end of the decade, the fellows might work nearly exclusively in only one of the training venues.

Dr. McIntosh required that fellow recruitment occur primarily through the Divisional office. On the first schedule the following appeared: "No additional commitments for fellowship support can be made without the approval of Dr. McIntosh".

As noted in the previous chapter, the majority of the fellows had an obligatory commitment in the military due to the "doctor draft". Dr. McIntosh was able to have several trainees, including Drs. Jess Peter and Doug Zipes, carry out their military obligation at the Portsmouth Naval Hospital. This afforded an additional opportunity for clinical training in cardiology.

Dr. McIntosh was very supportive of research within the Division. In 1965, in collaboration with Dr. David Sabiston (Department of Surgery) and Dr. Madison Spach (Department of Pediatrics), he initiated an annual Spring Scientific Cardiovascular Symposium. Fellows and junior faculty presented the results of their investigations to two or more visiting scientists. This Symposium was well attended and continued on an annual basis for the next 25 years.

Members of the Duke Cardiology Division became major participants in the annual meetings of the American Heart Association and American College of Cardiology. Prior to each national meeting, the fellows underwent a careful critique of their presentations by the senior staff. These review sessions turned out to be an outstanding learning experience for the fellows.

Thus, by the end of the decade, the opportunities for training had expanded dramatically. The Program had nearly doubled in size. The national and international reputation as an outstanding academic Training Program became firmly established.

Table 1 Cardiology Fellows: 1960–69

Name	Institution Internship/Residency	Fellowship Dates	Clinical Category	Research	Initial Career	Subsequent Career
Bache, Robert J.	U. Minnesota Hosp.	1967–69*	G	B	A	A
Behar, Victor S.	Duke Medical Center	1965–67	G–IV	C	A	A, Ret
Bennett, William T. (Tyson)	Tulane	1968–70	G		P	P, Ret
Boineau, John P.	Georgetown Duke Medical Center	1964–65	G	B	A	A
Carpenter, Harry M.	Bowman Gray Duke Medical Center—CR	1967–68*	G		P	P, Dec
Carter, William H.	Bellevue Hosp., NYC Columbia Medical Center, NYC Duke Medical Center	1967–70	G		P	P, A
Cobb, Frederick R.	Duke Medical Center	1967–68	G	B	A	A, Dec
Cohen, Allan I.	Duke Medical Center	1961–62	G		P	P, Dec
Cox, Ronnie L.	Duke Medical Center	1963–65	G	B	P	P, Ret
Craig, Robert J.	Royal Adelaide Hosp., Australia	1965–66*	G		A	P, Ret
Curry, Charles L.	Reynolds Hosp, Winston-Salem Duke Medical Center	1968–70	G	B	A	A, Ret
Dalton, Frank M.	Duke Medical Center	1967–69	G–IV		P	P, Dec
Davidson, Robert M.	Bellevue Hosp., NYC Duke Medical Center	1969–71	G		P	P
Dixon, II, Henry B.	McGill University, Montreal, Canada	1964–65*	G		P	P, Ret
Douglas, John E.	U. Michigan Medical Center Duke Medical Center—CR	1964–65 1966–67	G–IV	B	A	A, Ret

Name	Institution Internship/Residency	Fellowship Dates	Clinical Category	Research	Initial Career	Subsequent Career
Dunaway, Marshall C.	Duke Medical Center	1966–67*	C	C	P	P
Entman, Mark L.	Johns Hopkins Duke Medical Center	1964–66	G	B	A	A
Gaddy, Robert E.	Duke Medical Center U. North Carolina	1964–65	G		P	P, Ret
Garrison, Glen E.	U. Virginia, Charlottesville	1963–65	G		A	A
Gebel, Peter P.	U. Pennsylvania	1965–66	G		P	P, Ret
Giamber, Samuel R.	U. Pittsburgh U. Pennsylvania	1969–70*	G		P	P
Ginn, William M.	U. Florida, Gainesville Duke Medical Center	1964–65	G		P	P, Ret
Hallal, F. Joseph	U. Pittsburgh Duke Medical Center	1969–70	G		P	P
Harley, Alexander	West End Hosp., England Bristol Royal Infirmary, England	1965–67*	G	B	A	A
Harper, James R. (Bud)	U. Florida, Gainesville Duke Medical Center	1966–67*	G		P	A
Harris, Charles W.	Duke Medical Center	1963–64	G		P	P
Hernandez, Rafael R.	Duke Medical Center	1960–62	G–IV	B	A	P, Dec
Holland, Warren F.	Emory—Grady	1968–70	G		P	P, Ret
Holloway, David H.	Duke Medical Center	1963–64 1966–67	G		P	P
Hunt, Noel C.	Vanderbilt Duke Medical Center	1966–68	G–IV	B	P	P, Dec

Name	Institution Internship/Residency	Fellowship Dates	Clinical Category	Research	Initial Career	Subsequent Career
Hurlburt, James C.	Duke Medical Center	1962–64	G		P	P, Ret
Hurst, Victor W.	Yale, New Haven—CR	1965–66*	G–IV	B	A	P, OMI, Ret
Ira, Jr., Gordon H.	Duke Medical Center / Duval Medical Center, Jacksonville	1961–63	G		P	P, Ret
Irons, Jr., George V.	Barnes—Washington University / Billings Hosp., U. Chicago	1964–66	G		P	P
Johnson, Livingston	U. Pennsylvania / Bowman Gray	1968–69	G		P	P, Dec
Kendall, M. Eugene	Duke Medical Center	1969–71	G–IV	C	A	P, Ret
Kioschos, John M. (Mike)	Heidelberg, Germany / U. Iowa Hosp.	1966–67*	IV	B	A	A, Ret, Dec
Kong, Yihong (Dave)	The First Army General Hosp., Taipei, Taiwan / Schupert Memorial Hosp., Shreveport	1962–67	G–IV	C	A	A, Ret
Linhart, Joseph W.	George Washington University / Duke Medical Center	1962–63*	IV	C	A	A, Ret
McCall, Benjamin W.	Duke Medical Center	1962–63*	IV	C	A	P, Ret
McGowan, Ronald L.	Harrisburgh General Hosp. / Mayo, Rochester, NY	1968–70	G		OM	A, P, Ret
Moles, Stanley S.	U. Florida, Gainesville	1963–64	IV		P	P
Morris, James J.	Duke Medical Center—CR	1960–63	G–IV	C	A	A, Ret, Dec
Peter, Robert H. (Jess)	Duke Medical Center	1964–65 1967–68	G–IV	C	A	A, Ret
Rackley, Charles E.	Duke Medical Center	1963–66*	IV	C	A	A

Name	Institution Internship/Residency	Fellowship Dates	Clinical Category	Research	Initial Career	Subsequent Career
Ramo, Barry W.	U. Chicago Hosp. & Clinics	1967–69	G–IV	B	A	P
Roberts, Jr., Stewart R.	Duke Medical Center	1961–62	O	C	P	A, Ret
Roman-Irizarry, Luis	Puerto Rico	1967–69	G		P	P
Rosati, Robert A.	Duke Medical Center	1969–71	G	C	A	A, P
Rotman, Michael	Duke Medical Center	1968–71	G	C	P	P, OMI, Ret
Ruffy, Jr., Alfred J.	USPHS Hosp., New Orleans Tulane, Charity Hosp., New Orleans	1969–71	G		A	A, Ret
Ruskin, Jerome	Duke Medical Center	1965–67	G	C	A	P, Ret
Rygorsky, Jerome E.	Bronx Municipal Hosp. Center Mass. General Hosp. Duke Medical Center—CR	1967–68 1969–70	G		P	P, Ret
Saunders, III, Wade H.	U. Pittsburgh	1969–71	G		P	P, Ret
Schaal, Stephen F. (Rick)	Duke Medical Center	1966–68	G	B	A	A, Ret
Schoonmaker, Fred W.	Duke Medical Center—CR	1965–67	G		A	P, Ret, Dec
Shelburne, Palmer F.	Duke Medical Center Mass. Memorial Hosp.	1960–62	G		P	P, Ret
Sumner, Robert G.	Duke Medical Center	1962–63	IV		P	P, Ret, Dec
Wagner, Galen S.	Duke Medical Center	1967–68 1969–70	G	B	A	A
Wallace, Andrew G.	Duke Medical Center—CR	1961, 63*	G	B	A	A, Ret
Walston, II, Abe	Duke Medical Center	1966–68	G	B	A	P, OMI

Name	Institution Internship/Residency	Fellowship Dates	Clinical Category	Research	Initial Career	Subsequent Career
Waxman, Menashe B.	Jewish General Hosp., Montreal, Canada U. Pennsylvania Mount Sinai, NYC	1967–70	G–IV	B	A	A
Weglicki, Willliam B.	George Washington University	1964–66	G	B	A	A
Whalen, Robert E.	Duke Medical Center—CR	1960–61	G–IV	B	A	A, Ret
Wright, Kinsman E. (Ted)	Boston City Hosp.—CR Duke Medical Center	1969–70*	G		A	P, Ret
Zeft, Howard J.	Duke Medical Center	1966–68	G–IV	C	A	P
Zipes, Douglas P.	Duke Medical Center	1966–68*	G	B	A	A

See "Explanation for Data Tables" following Chapter II.

CHAPTER IV

1970–79

This decade began with a change in leadership. Dr. Henry McIntosh left to become Chairman of the Department of Medicine at Baylor Medical Center in Houston, Texas. Dr. Wyngaarden appointed Dr. Andy Wallace as Chief of the Division of Cardiology. Although Dr. Orgain retained the title of Chief of the Cardiovascular Disease Service, Andy's responsibility for the entire Division was unambiguous.

Interestingly, a change in Cardiology leadership near the beginning of each future decade became an established pattern.

Andy's primary goal regarding the future direction of Cardiology, and specifically the Fellowship Training Program, was to foster scientific investigation. He made a major commitment to the support of basic science. To meet this goal, early in the decade he made two outstanding recruits: Dr. Robert Lefkowitz in receptor biology and Dr. Harold Strauss in electrophysiology. After participating in the Framingham Study Program, Dr. Pat McKee returned to Duke and began investigating the basic mechanisms of clotting. These three investigators quickly developed outstanding research programs. Later in the decade, basic electrophysiology was strengthened by the addition of Dr. Raymond Ideker whose primary interest was ventricular activation and cardiac mapping. Although Ray was a cardiac pathologist, his laboratory space and research funds came through Cardiology. In addition, Dr. David Shand, who became Chief of Clinical Pharmacology and a member of the Cardiology Division, studied basic mechanisms of a number of cardioactive drugs. I had established an animal research laboratory at the DVAH which was dedicated to studying the factors which control myocardial perfusion using a variety of animal models.

Therefore, the fellows had the opportunity to train in one of these basic laboratories within the Cardiology Division. In addition, several chose to work with investigators from the basic science departments. Thus, by the end of the decade, approximately 50 percent of the fellows became involved in basic cardiovascular research (Chapter IX).

In recruiting fellows, Andy gave preference to those who were interested in pursuing training in basic cardiovascular research. As a consequence of "dual training", a fellowship of three years in duration became commonplace. In scheduling the research time, the "earlier the better" was the preferred strategy.

The Clinical Electrophysiology Program grew from "infancy" to a "full-fledged adult" extremely rapidly. As described previously, the surgical treatment of WPW required the development of techniques for intracardiac mapping. The necessary sophisticated equipment in large measure was developed "in house" by Jackie Kassel. Dr. John Gallagher was appointed the Director of the Clinical Electrophysiology Laboratory. In addition to his training in electrophysiology at Duke, John learned the technique of HIS bundle

27

recording from Dr. Tony Damato in New York. The rapid development of new technology was successfully utilized to markedly expand both the clinical service and clinical research in electrophysiology. The Cardiology Division soon became known as one of the top programs for training in both basic and clinical electrophysiology.

In fact, one of the more successful training paradigms was for the fellow to spend one year in basic electrophysiology with either Drs. Harold Strauss or Ray Ideker followed by a year in clinical electrophysiology.

As the reputation of the Cardiology Division spread, a number of fellows were attracted from outside the continental United States (Chapter VIII). During this decade, 15 percent of the fellows were foreign—recruited primarily from either the "Mother country" or the other "colonies". In general, these physicians were outstanding. Most of them had prior training in general cardiology and concentrated on specific clinical and research areas. In addition, of prime importance: they arrived—stipend in hand.

The development of echocardiography fell almost entirely on the shoulders of Dr. Joe Kisslo. While at Yale, Joe had rudimentary training in echocardiography. When he arrived as a fellow, he found an echo machine in a closet in Dr. Orgain's office. This instrument had been used, briefly, by Dr. Bill Carter while he was a fellow and then abandoned. While functioning as a fellow in the Catheterization Laboratory, Joe developed the Echocardiographic Clinical Service—which he headed for the next 20 years. In collaboration with Dr. Olaf von Ramm in Bioengineering, they developed one of the early phased array 2-D echo instruments and achieved instant notoriety. In addition to providing an excellent clinical service, the Echocardiographic Laboratory became an important venue for training fellows in both basic and clinical echocardiographic techniques.

Responsibility for the Duke Heart Station was transferred from the Cardiovascular Disease Service to me. The photographic instruments were replaced by direct-writing machines and the Heart Station was made responsible for recording all ECGs within Duke Medical Center (DUMC) on a 24-hour/day basis. (The number of documented ECGs recorded increased from 26,000 to 52,000 the first year.) In addition, vectorcardiography, using the Frank lead system, was made available for clinical use. All ECGs were read by both the fellows and senior cardiologists on a rotational basis. Other noninvasive procedures, i.e., Holtor monitoring, treadmill exercise tests and phonocardiograms, remained within the Cardiovascular Disease Service. Later, these tests were transferred to the Echocardiography Laboratory which was re-christened Cardiac Diagnostic Unit (CDU).

Interestingly, Nuclear Cardiology was developed at DUMC by Dr. Robert Jones in the Department of Surgery. Initially, these studies were primarily related to clinical research. However, when the technology advanced to the point of providing reliable clinical measurements of ventricular function, it was necessary to form a clinical service. Dr. Jones was disinterested in administrating this service. Unfortunately, the negotiations between Drs. Wyngaarden and Charles Putman, who was being recruited as Chief of Radiology, resulted in the transfer of Nuclear Cardiology to Radiology where it has been ever since. Thus, Nuclear Cardiology, although performing a clinical support role, was never an integral part of the clinical research of the Cardiology Division. Fellows frequently rotated through Nuclear Cardiology, especially at the DVAH, and a few of them obtained a license to utilize radioactive materials, but Nuclear Cardiology did not play a key role in fellowship training.

The Cardiology Databank, supported by the MIRU and later the SCOR (Specialized Center of Research), expanded to include all patients undergoing cardiac catheterization. Dr. Bob Rosati assumed a major role in this endeavor. (Bob had started his fellowship in basic electrophysiology, and decided after five months that clinical decision analysis was a better calling. Other than attending conferences, his efforts in the Databank encompassed Bob's total training in clinical cardiology.) Developing the capabilities to capture a large volume of clinical data, as well as a mechanism to follow these patients at preset intervals, was an enormous undertaking. The task was successfully carried out. Thus, the Cardiology Division was in a position to study the natural history of coronary disease and to evaluate the potential of various therapeutic modalities. Since coronary artery by-pass surgery was begun in earnest by 1969, it became important to incorporate similar clinical data on these patients as well. Dr. Alan Bartel began this endeavor, which further expanded the capability of the Databank as an important patient care and research tool.

One of the unique features of the approach to collecting verifiable clinical data involved the formulation of clinical reports. Since the Databank was responsible for the clinical reporting of catheterization data, and later on results from the CDU, the validity of these reports was guaranteed since they had to be read and signed by a clinician. Thus, the Databank performed an important hospital function, and at the same time, made certain that the data collected were valid.

Another vital aspect of the Databank was the development of biostatistical techniques to evaluate large patient populations. Initially, simple subgroups analyses were used to test for significant differences. Later on, sophisticated multivariate analyses techniques were utilized and frequently developed by the Databank biostatisticians (Drs. Kerry Lee and Frank Harrell). This avenue of investigation formed the basis for the statistical techniques to implement large clinical trials in subsequent decades. The importance of their work in the development of the Databank cannot be over estimated. The Databank proved to be a fertile area for training fellows in clinical research.

Early in the decade, a change occurred in the concept that a given fellow might train almost exclusively within a given component of the Division. Examination of the clinical schedules clearly indicates that significant crossover from the Cardiac Catheterization Laboratory, the DVAH, and the Cardiovascular Disease Service began to be commonplace. The amount of clinical training and the specific rotations, however, were not stereotyped—many fellows finished the Program with a significant variation in the amount of their clinical training. The duration of the clinical training, in general, was two years, although many fellows remained an extra year, primarily to carry out research. By mid-decade, a three-year fellowship was standard.

In order to provide didactic material, Andy developed a new conference format. A Saturday morning seminar, modeled after Dr. Stead's "Sunday School", became an essential feature of the Training Program. Fellows were required at least once a year to present a topic in depth. If possible, this presentation would encompass their own research. These seminars were held in a small room in which seating was available for approximately 80 percent of the attendees. (It was always clear who had arrived late because they had to stand up.) The interaction at this conference was outstanding. The conference was followed by a presentation in cardiac pathology by Dr. Donald Hackel.

The "Cath Conference" (adult and pediatric cardiology and cardiac surgery) continued, but was not as well attended as it had been in the preceding decade.

Formal research presentations in the Division were carried out at a monthly dinner program in which two fellows or junior staff members presented their current research. An effort was made to go over research that was just beginning so that a real critique by the attendees could be given. The annual Spring Symposium was continued in the same format, i.e., two outside experts (usually a cardiologist and a cardiac surgeon) were invited to critique the research. In addition, the fellows were encouraged to present at national cardiology meetings. Their talks were critiqued at specific rehearsal sessions. These sessions had two important purposes. They served to allow the fellow to have an excellent critique prior to the national presentation. In addition, everyone in the Division became conversant with the content of the presentation and although rarely, if disagreements occurred, they could be adjudicated. For example, did we really want to present the surgical mortality in left main stenosis at a national meeting?

A notable event occurred when Dr. George Cooper won the newly constituted Katz Award for Young Investigators at the American Heart Association annual meeting. George carried out studies to define the relationship between myocardial mechanics and oxygen consumption.

By mid-decade, Andy Wallace became quite interested in cardiac rehabilitation and prevention. In 1976, he decided to take a sabbatical leave to develop a program at Duke. DUPAC (Duke University Preventative Approach to Cardiology) was born. As was uniformly the case with Andy's endeavors, within a few years, the Program was widely recognized and became an important clinical function of the Division. Although initially housed in borrowed space, in conjunction with the Department of Athletics, the Finch Yeager Building was constructed and became the home for DUPAC. In addition to providing an outstanding clinical service, the patients became an important source for the development of clinical research, including studies of exercise physiology and clinical follow-up of various treatment modalities. A number of fellows became involved in research carried out in the DUPAC venue.

An unexpected and extremely worthwhile situation resulted from this endeavor: a number of the participants were wealthy. For example, Mr. David Thomas (Wendy's) came to the Program. As a consequence, the Thomas Center at the Fuqua School of Business became a reality. The Stedman Nutrition Center also had its origin from personal interaction at DUPAC with Mr. David Stedman.

In order to concentrate on the development of DUPAC, Andy appointed Galen Wagner as the acting Division Chief. Although the job description was somewhat unclear, Galen was responsible for the day-by-day activity of the Division—but major decisions regarding faculty, etc., were continued to be made by Andy. Administration of the Fellowship Program fell in large measure under Galen's purview. Thus, Galen became the first non-division chief to direct the Cardiology Training Program. Since he was keenly interested in this endeavor, he made a major effort to dramatically improve the Program. Of prime importance was the development of strategies to recruit the best fellows possible. There are numerous examples of outstanding fellows who chose Duke primarily because of Galen's efforts. Under his direction, the size of the Program increased dramatically. At that time, the Fellowship Training Program had to "stand on its own bottom" financially. The potential problems with adequate funding resulted in a number of heated discussions between Andy and Galen regarding the number of fellows to be recruited. In fact, this continual disagreement regarding the size of the Program became a significant issue which resulted in the appointment of Dr. Ed Pritchett as Program Director in 1979. Galen went on to other endeavors, but clearly left an indelible imprint on the Fellow Training Program.

The Training Program continued to expand and, as noted previously, the majority of the fellows signed up for three years. The usual recruitment plan required that the fellows were chosen primarily to be involved in a clinical or research laboratory. Thus, the area of their particular interest was known prior to the beginning of their fellowship training. Significant crossover occurred, but this approach provided trainees for each of the basic and clinical research laboratories. Although every aspect of cardiology was available in specific rotations, the fellows still could finish the clinical training without completing a "core curriculum".

The period 1970–79 was an outstanding time of maturing for the Fellowship Program. So much so, that by any yardstick, it became one of the best Programs in the country for the training of academic cardiologists.

Table 1 Cardiology Fellows: 1970–79

Name	Institution Internship/Residency	Fellowship Dates	Clinical Category	Research	Initial Career	Subsequent Career
Alexander, R. Wayne	Duke Medical Center U. Washington	1974–76*	G	B	A	A
Aronson, Ronald S.	Johns Hopkins	1973–75*	G	B	A	A, P, OMI
Baker, John T.	Duke Medical Center	1973–75	G		A	P, Ret
Bartel, Alan G.	U. Miami Duke Medical Center	1970–72	G-IV	C	A	P
Bashore, Thomas M.	U. North Carolina	1975–77	G-IV	C	A	P, A
Benditt, David G.	U. Manitoba, Canada	1975–78	G-EP	B	A	A
Bethea, Charles F.	Duke Medical Center	1972–73 1974–75	G		P	P
Bilbro, Robert H.	Parkland—UTSW U. North Carolina	1971–72	G		P	P, Ret
Bramlet, Dean A.	U. Minnesota	1979–81	G		P	P
Brenner, Alan S. (Sandy)	Duke Medical Center	1971–73	G-IV		P	P, Ret
Brewer, David L.	U. Oklahoma Duke Medical Center—CR	1971–72	G-IV		A	P
Burks, John M.	UCSF	1975–77	G		P	P
Busch, Calvert R.	Milwaukee County Hosp.	1975–76*	G		P	P
Calder, Joseph R.	U. Iowa Hospitals & Clinics	1973–75	G-IV		P	P, Ret, Dec
Campbell, Ronald W. F.	New Castle General Hosp., England	1975–76*	EP	C	A	A, Dec
Colvard,Jr., M. Clark	Baroness Erlanger Hosp., Chattanooga U. Miami	1970–72	G		P	P

Name	Institution Internship/Residency	Fellowship Dates	Clinical Category	Research	Initial Career	Subsequent Career
Conley, Jr., Martin J.	Duke Medical Center	1975–78 1980–91*	G	C	P	P
Conn, Eric H.	Yale, New Haven	1979–81	G		A	P
Cooper, IV, George	U. Hosp., Cleveland	1973–75*	G	B	A	A
Cope, Geoffrey D. (Jeff) •	Royal North Shore Hosp., Sydney, Australia Launceston Gen. Hosp., Launceston, Australia Royal Perth Hosp., Perth, W. Australia	1974–75*	NIV	C	P	P
Davis, Dwight	Boston University Medical Center	1978–81	G–EP	B	A	A
Dillon, Michael C.	Duke Medical Center—CR	1978–80	G		P	P
Dixon, Jr., John H.	Vanderbilt—CR	1975–77	G		P	P, A
Dohrmann, Mary L.	Missouri Health Sciences Center	1977–79	G–EP		OM	A, P, A
Dugan, Fortune A. (Jim)	Tulane, Charity Hosp., New Orleans	1973–75	G–IV		A	P
Fauntleroy, Jr., Thomas W.	Duke Medical Center	1971–74	G		P	P, Ret
Ferguson, Earl W.	U. Texas, Galveston Duke Medical Center	1973–75	G	B	A	OM (A), OMI, P
Fraker, Jr., Theodore D.	The Ohio State University	1976–79	G	C	A	A
Gallagher, John J.	Duke Medical Center	1972–74*	G–EP	C	A	P
German, Lawrence D.	Strong Memorial Hosp., Rochester, NY	1979–81	G–EP	B	A	P, Dec
Gibbons, Raymond J.	Mass. General Hosp.	1978–81	G	C	A	A
Gilbert, Brian W.	U. Toronto, Canada Duke Medical Center	1975–76*	NIV	C	A	A

Name	Institution Internship/Residency	Fellowship Dates	Clinical Category	Research	Initial Career	Subsequent Career
Gilbert, David B.	Barnes—Washington University Duke Medical Center	1970–72	G	B	A	P
Gilbert, Marcel R.	Hosp. St. Sacrement, Quebec, Canada Montpellier, France	1971–73*	G	C	A	A
Grant, Augustus O. (Gus)	Hahnemann Medical College, Philadelphia U. Manitoba, Canada	1977–80	G-EP	B	A	A
Green, Larry S.	Duke Medical Center Utah Medical Center—CR	1975–76*	G	B	A	A, P, A
Grove, David D.	Cleveland Metropolitan Gen. Hosp.—CR	1977–80	G	B	P	P, Ret
Guarnieri, Thomas	Johns Hopkins—CR	1979–82	G-EP	B	A	P
Habersberger, Peter G.	Alfred Hosp., Melbourne, Australia	1972–73*	G		P	P
Hammill, Stephen C.	U. Colorado	1978–81*	G-EP	C	A	A
Handel, Franklin	The Ohio State University	1979–83	G	B	P	P
Harris, Phillip J.	Royal Prince Alfred Hosp, Sydney, Australia	1977–79*	G	C	A	A
Harrison, David G.	Duke Medical Center	1977–79	G		P	A
Hartman, Carl W.	Duke Medical Center	1973–75	G		A	P
Hindman, Michael C.	Duke Medical Center—CR	1977–79	G-IV	B	A	P, Ret
Hirshfeld, Jr., John W.	Yale, New Haven	1973–74*	IV		A	A
Irvin, Robert G.	U. Virginia, Charlottesville MUSC, Charleston	1975–77	G	B	A	P, Ret
Johnson, Benjamin D.	Wilford Hall Medical Center, Lackland AFB	1970–72	G		P	P
Juk, Jr., S. Stanley	U. Alabama Hosp. Clinic	1973–75	G-IV		P	P

Name	Institution Internship/Residency	Fellowship Dates	Clinical Category	Research	Initial Career	Subsequent Career
Kent, Richard S.	Peter Bent Brigham Stanford U. Hosp.	1978–81	G	B	A	OMI
Kerr, Charles R.	Vancouver General Hosp., Canada Hammersmith Hosp., Brompton Hosp., London, England	1979–81*	EP	B	A	A
Kisslo, Joseph A.	Hahnemann University Hosp., Philadelphia Yale, New Haven	1972–74	G–IV	C	A	A
Klein, George J.	Suny Brook, Toronto, Canada St. Paul's Hosp., Vancouver, Canada	1977–79*	EP	B	A	A
Lester, Robert M.	Duke Medical Center	1976–79*	G–NIV	C	A	P, OMI
Lieppe, William M.	SUNY, Syracuse, NY	1975–78	G–NIV	C	A	P
Low, Lip Ping	U. Singapore	1972*	IV		P	A, P
Mahony, Cheryl	Duke Medical Center	1979–82	G	B	A	P, Ret
Margolis, James R.	Barnes—Washington University	1972–74	G–IV	C	A	P
Mays, Jr., Arthur E. •	SUNY—Buffalo	1979–81*	G	B	P	P
McEwan, Patricia M.	Toronto Western Hosp., Canada	1978–79*	NIV	C	A	A, P
McGrew, III, Frank A.	U. Hosp., Cleveland	1974–76	G		P	P
McNeer, James F. (Fred)	Duke Medical Center	1972–73 1976–77	G	C	A	P
Miller, Hugh C.	Edinburgh Royal Infirmary, Scotland Brompton Hosp., London, England	1973–74*	G	B	A	A, Ret
Mittler, Brant S.	Baylor Affiliated Hosp., Houston Baltimore City Hosp.	1974–76	G	C	P	P, O
Morris, Kenneth G.	The Ohio State University	1976–78	G–NIV	C	A	A

Name	Institution Internship/Residency	Fellowship Dates	Clinical Category	Research	Initial Career	Subsequent Career
Nichol, Peter M.	U. Western Ontario, Canada — CR	1975–76*	NIV	C	A	P, Ret
Oelrich, William L.	Baylor Affiliated Hosp., Houston	1974–76	G		P	P
Palmeri, Sebastian T.	Duke Medical Center	1978–80	G	C	A	P, A
Parker, John P.	The Ohio State University	1976–79	G	B	P	P
Port, Steven C.	Mount Sinai, NYC	1975–79	G–NIV	C	A	A, P
Pritchett, Edward L. C.	University Hosp., Columbus, OH	1974–76	G–EP	C	A	A, OMI
Pryor, David B.	Pennsylvania Hosp., Philadelphia	1979–82	G	C	A	A, OMI
Prystowsky, Eric N.	Mount Sinai, NYC	1976–79	G–EP	B	A	A, P
Reed, John B.	Duke Medical Center	1972–74	G–IV		A	P
Reinhart, Richard A. (Rick)	Duke Medical Center	1973–74 1979–80*	G		P	A, P, A, P
Reiter, Michael J.	Parkland — UTSW	1978–82	G–EP	C	A	A
Rhodes, Charles M.	Duke Medical Center	1977–79	G		OMI	P
Richter, Henry S.	Bellevue Hosp., NYC Duke Medical Center	1971–73	G		P	P
Rivas, Frank	St. Louis University — CR	1973–75*	G	B	A	A, P
Rogers, Garrett L.	Duke Medical Center	1976–78	G		P	P, A, P
Rubenstein, Carl J.	Duke Medical Center	1970–72*	G	B	A	P
Russell, John H.	U. Pennsylvania — CR	1970–71*	G		P	P, Ret
Scallion, Ralph M.	Case Western Reserve	1976–78	G–NIV	C	A	OMI, P.
Schocken, Douglas D.	Duke Medical Center	1978–81*	G	B	A	A
Silverstein, Burton V.	U. Pennsylvania	1975–77	G		P	P

Name	Institution Internship/Residency	Fellowship Dates	Clinical Category	Research	Initial Career	Subsequent Career
Simon, Arthur B.	Kings County Hosp., Brooklyn Michael Reese Hosp.	1970–72	G		P	P, Ret
Slagle, Richard C.	U. Oklahoma Duke Medical Center	1971–73	G-IV		P	P
Slosky, David A.	Duke Medical Center	1978–81	G	C	P	P, A
Smith, Warren M.	Auckland Hosp., New Zealand Middlemore Hosp., New Zealand	1978–79*	G-EP	B	A	P
Spencer, III, William H.	Johns Hopkins Duke Medical Center	1970–72	G		P	P, A
Stack, Richard S.	Wayne State University—CR	1979–82	G-NIV	B	A	A, OMI
Starr, John W.	Duke Medical Center	1973–75 1976–77	G	C	P	P
Stewart, James A.	Montreal General Hosp., Canada	1978–80*	NIV	C	A	A
Stiles, Gary L.	Vanderbilt	1978–81	G	B	A	A, OMI
Svenson, Robert H.	U. Chicago Hosp. & Clinics	1972–75	G-IV	C	P	P
Swain, Judith L.	Duke Medical Center	1976–80	G	B	A	A
Ticzon, Andres R.	Southside Hosp., Pittsburgh U. Minnesota	1971–73*	G-EP	B	P	P, Ret
Tonkin, Andrew M.	Royal Melbourne Hosp., Australia	1973–75*	G-EP	C	A	A
Turner, Harrison D.	Parkland—UTSW U. North Carolina	1976–78	G		P	P
Tysinger, John R.	George Washington University	1977–78*	G		P	P

Name	Institution Internship/Residency	Fellowship Dates	Clinical Category	Research	Initial Career	Subsequent Career
Upton, Mark T.	New York Hosp., NYC Mary Hitchcock Memorial Hosp., Hanover, NH	1977–79*	G–NIV	C	P	P
Vranian, Robert B.	Parkland—UTSW U. North Carolina	1976–78	G		P	P
Warner, Robert A.	Upstate, Syracuse, NY	1972–75	G	C	A	A, Ret, OMI
Warren, Stafford G.	U. Hosp., Cleveland	1972–74	G		P	P
Waugh, Robert A.	U. Pennsylvania	1970–72*	G	B	P	A
Wenger, Thomas L.	Harlem Hosp., NYC Duke Medical Center	1975–78	G	B	OMI	OMI
Williams, R. Sanders (Sandy)	Mass. General Hosp.	1977–80	G	B	A	A
Wise, Neil K. (Kent)	U. Illinois Hosp., Chicago	1977–80	G–NIV	C	P	P
Yatteau, Ronald F.	MCV, Richmond Wilford Hall Medical Center, Lackland AFB	1970–72	G		P	P

See "Explanataion for Data Tables" following Chapter II.

CHAPTER V

1980–89

In 1980, a momentous occasion occurred at Duke Medical Center: Duke Hospital North was occupied. In spite of significant opposition, Chancellor William Anlyan went out on a "very narrow limb" and had the new structure built. Prior to this time, growth of the clinical enterprise had been constrained by medieval type architecture constructed in the 1930s: beautiful to look at, but an efficient hospital—no!

Cardiology successfully negotiated for considerable space on the seventh floor of the new structure; including two cardiac catheterization laboratories for routine diagnostic cases and an electrophysiology catheterization laboratory adjacent to the Cardiac Care Unit (CCU). The Heart Station was assigned considerable excess space which over the next few years was used to house multiple cardiology functions. Office space was provided for a number of clinicians. (In fact, Cardiology was the only medical subspecialty with significant office space in Duke North.) The CCU contained eight acute beds and four step-down beds. In addition, two non-acute wards having 32 beds each were assigned primarily to Cardiology. Thus, as far as "real estate" was concerned, Cardiology was in a position to significantly expand the inpatient clinical service.

In 1980, Dr. Roscoe (Ike) Robinson resigned as Hospital Director to become Chancellor at Vanderbilt and Dr. Andy Wallace decided to try his hand at hospital administration. Dr. Wyngaarden asked me to lead the Cardiology Division in early 1981.

After discussing the future direction of the Division with the faculty, we began an initiative to dramatically increase both the size and scope of the clinical service. Ancillary facilities were excellent and the hospital beds underutilized. Thus, the opportunity for significant growth in inpatient services was clearly available.

Although coronary bypass surgery had been available at Duke for nearly a decade, the yearly number of operations had increased only moderately. At a meeting with Dr. David Sabiston and the cardiovascular surgeons, I proposed that Cardiology take the initiative to markedly increase the number of patients referred for cardiac surgery. Although the surgeons were quite receptive to this notion, they adopted a "wait and see" attitude.

As outlined below, a number of salient factors occurred almost simultaneously, which allowed a complete redirection in the modalities available for the treatment of patients with acute coronary syndromes. The Cardiology Division, in large measure, quickly became a national leader in this revolution.

At this time, both nationally and at Duke, there was considerable interest in developing strategies to limit the size of myocardial infarction in patients with acute coronary occlusion. Multiple approaches were tried to protect the ischemic myocardium. However, the results were unimpressive. The possibility of reperfusion, using either thrombolytic agents or mechanical intervention, was in its infancy. Several of the cardiac surgeons at Duke were among the first to demonstrate the efficacy of bypass surgery carried out during the peri-infarct period. However, the real "breakthrough" occurred with the development of functional thrombolytic agents.

Dr. Rob Califf, after finishing a two-year cardiology fellowship, became Director of the CCU in 1983. He immediately initiated a series of trials to utilize and test thrombolytic agents in patients with acute myocardial infarction. These studies, carried out under the rubric of TAMI (Thrombolysis in Acute Myocardial Infarction), achieved considerable notoriety. The number of patients with acute myocardial infarction referred for reperfusion therapy dramatically increased, resulting in an expansion in the number of acute CCU beds to 16.

One of the issues that had to be dealt with was effecting a change in the referral system to Cardiology. The Cardiovascular Disease Service provided an outstanding cardiac consultation service. However, many physicians who referred patients had already made the decision that cardiac catheterization was indicated. Thus, their patients did not need a detailed consultation. Dr. Harry Phillips, who had been Chief of the Cardiac Catheterization Laboratory at the DVAH, developed a service at Duke to handle these patients. Soon he was joined by Drs. Rob Califf and Jess Peter and the PCP Service (Phillips, Califf and Peter) was created. Within short order, the number of patients referred to Cardiology markedly increased. When Dr. Vic Behar joined the group, the CAD Service (Cardiology at Duke) came into being. Membership in the CAD Service increased rapidly in order to care for the large influx of patients.

The final component of the change in the direction of the clinical service occurred with the development of Interventional Cardiology. Although a few angioplasties had been performed at Duke prior to 1981, there was little interest in expanding this program. Dr. John Simpson, a former house officer at Duke, had developed innovative technology to guide the catheters during angioplasty. He visited the institution and agreed to help with the development of the interventional program.

A major stimulus to the development of Interventional Cardiology resulted from a very successful angioplasty in a patient with acute myocardial infarction. In 1982 a patient, one of my close friends, arrived in the Emergency Room in cardiogenic shock and complete heart block approximately one hour after the onset of chest pain. Jess Peter successfully opened the right coronary artery; the patient not only survived, but also had essentially normal ventricular function. Lesson learned: The heart works better when adequately perfused.

In 1983, Dr. Richard Stack, who had recently finished fellowship training and was Director of the CCU at the DVAH, became Chief of the Interventional Program. There were two significant obstacles which had to be overcome before significant development could begin: 1) obtain adequate laboratory space and 2) negotiate appropriate surgical backup.

By that time, the two existing diagnostic catheterization laboratories were heavily utilized and additional space was desperately needed. Magnanimously, Dr. Charles Putman, (Chief of Radiology) agreed to solve the first problem. Space and equipment for two interventional catheterization laboratories were provided on the first floor of Duke North. Dr. David Sabiston (Chief of Surgery) agreed to provide surgical backup: a decision of major importance. (At this time in many academic institutions, angioplasty programs were throttled because of the unwillingness of the cardiovascular surgeons to provide this service.)

The combination of a creative spark in developing new technology by Dr. Richard Stack and his co-workers, along with the dramatic influx of patients with acute my-ocardial infarction for angioplasty, combined so that the growth of this service was as-tronomical. Later in the decade, the Program expanded to include interventional ap-proaches to peripheral vascular disease.

One of the limiting factors was the development of a transport system to handle this large influx of cardiology patients. The concept of utilizing a helicopter for this task was envisioned. Previously, helicopters had been employed in a few medical centers primarily to transport accident victims, but the use for acute cardiac patients was unique. Although the "feasibility studies" by the hospital administration indicated that utilization would be minimal, the first month that Life Flight functioned, the projected number of flights for the entire year was exceeded. (So much for feasibility studies.) Approximately 70 percent of the patients transported by helicopter arrived for treat-ment of acute myocardial infarction.

When Life Flight was initiated, a senior cardiologist was always a member of the flight team. In developing the program, each referral center designated a location for the helicopter to land. However, on several occasions, access to the patient from this site was blocked. A notable occasion occurred one night when the helicopter landed on the wrong side of an eight-foot high chain-link fence topped with barbed wire. The gate was locked. No one appeared immediately to solve the problem. Richard Stack, wearing *Ninjutsu* footwear, scaled the fence and found the appropriate individual to unlock the gate.

Although helicopter transportation was associated with potential mishaps, in gen-eral, very few untoward events occurred. On one occasion, due to mechanical failure, the helicopter had to be landed emergently in a farm field. Luckily, no one was hurt. The patient being transported was asked about the incident. He frowned and mum-bled: "That air plane ride cured my chest pain, but that trip was somewhat bumpy".

The changes in the immediate treatment of patients with acute myocardial infarc-tion had a profound positive effect on the mortality and morbidity of these patients. The strategies employed at Duke not only were successful for the patients in the refer-ral area in North Carolina, but also were emulated throughout the rest of the country.

Dr. Tom Bashore returned to Duke in 1985 as Director of the Diagnostic Catheter-ization Laboratory. Under his tutelage, the administrative structure was markedly streamlined and an additional catheterization laboratory was added. Tom's primary clinical interest, valvular and congenital heart disease, led to the development of catheter-induced valvuloplasty. In addition, he organized a robust clinical service to follow this cadre of patients.

The number of diagnostic cardiac catheterizations, interventional procedures and coronary bypass operations dramatically increased over the decade: 1900 to 4200, 25 to 1300, and 400 to 950, respectively.

As a secondary but positive feature, the professional fees collected from these en-deavors enabled a very significant growth in the Cardiology Division as well as the rest of the Department of Medicine. The financial effects on DUMC were also profound. Monies from the technical fees were used to finish constructing Duke North (two floors) so that all of the inpatient services were moved from Duke South. In fact, much of the debt incurred in building Duke North was retired. In truth, Cardiology "saved the day".

The significant growth and redirection of the clinical cardiology service had a profound impact on the fellowship. The size of the Program significantly increased. The need for additional fellows also resulted from the decision to change the Program to a three-year requirement in which 18 months was spent in more or less standard clinical rotations and 18 months in research. This strategy guaranteed that each fellow would have specific research training. As in the past, basic investigation in cardiovascular disease processes was the major thrust of the research training. The strategy to recruit fellows to a specific laboratory became a universal plan. In many cases, they began research training at the beginning of their fellowship.

In order to be successful, the ability of a fellow to change research objectives had to be available. For example, Dr. Gary Stiles, recruited to work with Dr. Fred Cobb in clinical studies of congestive heart failure, had a change of interest. After meeting with Dr. Bob Lefkowitz, he plotted a new direction: receptor biology.

A second significant new approach to training occurred with the development of an 18 month core curriculum. Interestingly enough, the initial schedule was devised at one of the Wednesday night research dinner meetings. Deliberations between Dr. Ed Pritchett and I resulted in a prototype schedule being inscribed on a paper napkin (Figure). This schedule generally was followed throughout the decade.

A very significant issue occurred when a number of fellows expressed a desire to train in interventional cardiology. For the first year of the Program, only one fellow, Dr. Tom Hinohara was trained. (His call schedule was twenty-four hours a day, seven days a week for the entire year.) In order to be certain that the fellows who participated in interventional techniques would be thoroughly trained, the number was limited to two fellows per year and expanded to four years in length.

This decision to limit the number of interventional trainees created considerable discord among the fellows. Several of the fellows who desired interventional training were sent to various other laboratories throughout the United States and Canada. With rare exceptions, everyone who wanted to have interventional training achieved their goal. However, those trained at Duke had a wealth of experience in both interventional technology and research. This decision to limit the number of fellows receiving in-depth interventional training was unique among cardiology training programs. Defining a rigorous curriculum only occurred nationally with the belated institution of the interventional board requirements in 1999 (Chapter XII).

Dr. Ed Pritchett continued as the Program Director and dealt with the knotty problems associated with participating in the National Fellow Match (Chapter VIII). A unique feature of the matching program: interventional fellows were matched in a separate group. The match became a significant impediment to the strategy of recruiting fellows into specific research environments. However, Ed worked extremely hard—and by and large made the best of a bad situation. In 1988, Dr. Gary Stiles became Program Director. The administrative aspects of the Training Program were very ably carried out by Mollie Sykes and later by Mary Forrest.

A significant number of new basic science laboratories within Cardiology became available for fellowship training. Although Dr. David Shand had left, the other laboratories present in the previous decade continued. A number of investigators developed new basic science laboratories: Drs. Judy Swain, Sandy Williams, Fred Cobb, Gus

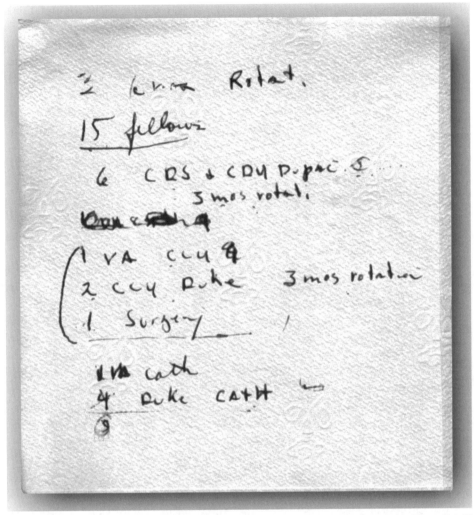

Figure The schedule for the first (1983) 18-month core curriculum was "inscribed" on a paper napkin and preserved for posterity by Ed Pritchett.

Grant, Gary Stiles, Frank Starmer and Richard Stack. Each of these laboratories was significantly involved with training of the fellows.

The DUPAC Program was expanded and new facilities opened under the rubric of the Center for Living. Both cardiac rehabilitation and prevention were primary goals. After Dr. Andy Wallace left to become Chancellor at Dartmouth, Dr. Fred Cobb assumed the responsibility of directing the Program. Soon it became a locus for fellowship training in both rehabilitation and exercise physiology.

Early in the decade, the Databank which had been funded in large measure through NHI grants (MIRU and later SCOR) radically changed. Funding from the SCOR was no longer available and the continual accruing of patient data had to be funded out of Divisional resources. Dr. Bob Rosati began working with Dr. Walter Kempner in the Rice Diet Program and Frank Starmer left to carry out research in basic electrophysiology. Drs. Rob Califf and David Pryor took on the responsibility for the development and funding of the Databank. David's primary role was to develop the computational technology as well as to foster the outcomes research. Rob's primary function was the development of clinical trials. The biostatistical group became internationally known for their work in data management. A large number of fellows decided to carry out their research in this fertile environment. In order to meet the financial needs, soon it became obvious that clinical trials would be the primary source of funds. Thus, by the end of the decade, clinical trials became by far the largest component of the Databank.

Initially, the Electrophysiology Service continued to develop new technology, e.g., catheter-based ablation. However, when Dr. Gallagher left, the innovative aspects of the program suffered. Led by Drs. Larry German, Eric Prystowsky (briefly) and Marcus Wharton, the Service stayed abreast of the developments in modern technology, but did not lead the field. The patient volume expanded considerably. An increasing number of fellows received training in clinical electrophysiology. The concept of spending a year in basic electrophysiology prior to clinical training was continued, although it was not as universal as in the previous decade.

Housed in the CDU, the echocardiographic program remained under the tutelage of Dr. Joe Kisslo and continued to stay at the forefront of developing technology, e.g., color flow Doppler. In collaboration with the congenital heart disease surgeons, Joe initiated studies in the operating room to define ventricular function and intracardiac shunts using direct echocardiographic measurements. The CDU provided the opportunity for a number of fellows to carry out clinical research projects.

The conference schedules continued as in the previous decade with the Saturday morning seminars and the monthly research meetings. These were extremely well attended and continued to provide a cohesive venue for interaction with fellows and faculty. Under the aegis of the Fellows Society, in 1982, the yearly Orgain Symposium was established to provide an avenue for interaction with fellow alumni.

The importance of presentations by the fellows became a major goal of the Division. Considerable effort was spent in tutoring the fellows' presentations so that they could function on a national stage. The number of presentations from the Division at both the American Heart Association and American College of Cardiology annual meetings were consistently among the top. In addition, the fellows were required not to stop with the submission of an abstract, but to complete and publish their work; thus, enforcing the academic mission of the Training Program.

This decade can be characterized as a period of rapid growth in size and direction of the Cardiology Division and the Fellowship Program. The dramatic expansion of the clinical service, especially the treatment of patients with acute myocardial infarction, along with the remarkable growth of the Interventional Program, markedly changed the nature of the clinical training. The Program became a standard three-year commitment with a major research component being mandatory.

The primary emphasis remained unchanged: prepare the fellows for academic careers in Cardiology.

Table 1 Cardiology Fellows: 1980–89

Name	Institution Internship/Residency	Fellowship Dates	Clinical Category	Research	Initial Career	Subsequent Career
Adamick, Richard D.	Stanford	1983–86	G	B	P	P
Allen, Mary F. Maturi	U. Maryland	1984–86*	G	B	P	P
Annex, Brian H.	Tufts, Boston	1988–92*	G	B	A	A
Barber, Michael J.	U. Virginia, Charlottesville	1987–90	G	B	A	P
Bardy, Gust H.	Northwestern	1980–83	G–EP	B	A	A, OMI
Barrington, William W.	Presbyterian Hosp., Pittsburgh	1987–91	G–EP	B	A	A
Bauman, Robert P.	Wayne State University	1984–88	G–IC	B	A	P
Beere, Polly A.	Duke Medical Center	1989–92	G	C	A	OMI, O
Belkin, Robert N.	New York Hosp., NYC	1983–86	G	C	A	A, P
Bellinger, Raye L.	USAF Medical Center., Keesler AFB	1985–87	G–IC		OM	P
Bengtson, James R.	U. Mass. Medical Center	1986–88	G	C	A	P
Berry, Jonathan J.	Duke Medical Center	1986–89*	G	B	P	P
Blackshear, Joseph L.	Hennepin County, Minneapolis	1984–86*	G	C	P	P
Broughton, Archer	H.S. Royal Prince Alfred Hosp., Australia	1981–83*	EP	B	P	P
Buller, Christopher E.	U. Toronto, Canada U. British Columbia, Canada	1989–91*	IC	C	A	A
Califf, Robert M.	UCSF Duke Medical Center	1980–82	G	C	A	A
Campbell, Paul T.	Duke Medical Center	1988–92	G	B	P	P
Carlson, Eric B.	MCV, Richmond	1983–86	G–IC	C	A	P
Chambers, David E.	Duke Medical Center	1989–92	G	B	P	P

Name	Institution Internship/Residency	Fellowship Dates	Clinical Category	Research	Initial Career	Subsequent Career
Chapman, Gregory D.	New York Hosp., NYC	1988–92	G–IC	B	A	A, P
Chen, Peng-Sheng	Parkland—UTSW	1984–88	G–EP	B	A	A
Chu, A. Alan	Duke Medical Center	1982–85	G	B	A	P
Clair, Walter K.	Brigham & Women's Hosp.—CR	1989–93	G–EP	C	P	P, A
Colavita, Paul G.	Georgetown	1982–85	G–EP	B	A	P
Collins, Gary J.	Wright-Patterson AFB Medical Center	1985–87*	IC		OM	P
Culp, Stephen C.	Duke Medical Center	1989–92	G–IC	B	A	P
Curtis, Ann B.	Presbyterian Hosp., NYC	1982–86	G–EP	B	A	A
Daubert, James P.	Duke Medical Center—CR	1989–92	G–EP	B	A	A
Davidson, Charles J.	Northwestern	1985–88	G–IC	C	A	A
Denning, Stephen M.	U. Chicago	1983–86	G	B	A	P
Deweese, Gary K.	Duke Medical Center	1989–91	G		P	P
Durand, John L.	U. Texas, San Antonio	1980–82	G	C	P	P
Elion, Jon L.	U. Wisconsin	1980–83	G	B	A	A, OMI
Ellenbogen, Kenneth A.	Johns Hopkins	1983–86	G–EP	C	A	A
Fananapazir, Lameh	Royal Infirmary, Edinburgh, Scotland	1986–87*	EP	C	A	A, P
Fedor, John M.	Duke Medical Center	1980–83	G	B	A	P
Feneley, Michael P. •	St. Vincent's Hosp., Sydney, Australia	1985–87*	NIV	C	A	A
Fetters, Julie K.	Duke Medical Center	1989–92	G	B	A	P
Fortin, Donald F.	Parkland—UTSW—CR	1988–91	G–IC	C	A	OMI
Frid, David J.	U. Mass. Medical Center	1988–91*	G	C	A	A, P, OMI
Gammon, Roger S.	Parkland—UTSW—CR	1988–92	G–IC	B	P	P

Name	Institution Internship/Residency	Fellowship Dates	Clinical Category	Research	Initial Career	Subsequent Career
Gilliam, III, F. Roosevelt (Rosie)	Duke Medical Center	1985–88	G–EP	B	A	P, A, P
Granger, Christopher B.	U. Colorado—CR	1988–90	G	C	A	A
Greenfield, Ruth Ann	Duke Medical Center	1988–91	G–EP	C	A	A
Greer, G. Stephen	U. Hosp., Little Rock	1984–87	G–EP	C	P	P
Grierson, David S.	Duke Medical Center	1981–84	G–IV	B	A	P
Griffen, III, D. Leonard	National Naval Medical Center, Bethesda	1989–90*	NIV	C	P	P
Gurbel, Paul A.	Duke Medical Center—CR	1987–88 1989–91	G–IC	C	A	P
Hamilton, Karen K.	Johns Hopkins	1982–85	G	B	A	P, A
Harding, Michael B.	Vanderbilt	1988–91*	G	C	P	P
Harrison, J. Kevin	Johns Hopkins	1988–90	G–IV	C	A	A
Hassel, C. David	U. Florida, Gainesville	1982–84	G	C	P	P
Hassett, M. Alycia	Emory—Grady	1981–84	G	B	A	P
Heard, Maurice E. (Tripp)	Johns Hopkins	1987–90	G–EP	C	A	P
Heinle, Shelia A.	Duke Medical Center	1989–91	G–NIV	C	A	A, P
Heinsimer, James A.	Dartmouth Affiliated Hosp.	1981–84	G	B	A	A, P, A
Henke, Elizabeth R.	U. Hosp. of Wales U. North Carolina	1984–86*	G		P	P
Hermiller, James B.	National Naval Medical Center, Bethesda—CR	1989–92	G–IV	C	P	P
Hettleman, Bruce D.	Duke Medical Center	1980–83	G–REH	C	A	A
Higginbotham, Michael B.	Royal Melbourne Hosp., Australia	1981–83*	G	C	A	A, P
Himmelstein, Stevan I.	Duke Medical Center	1985–88	G	B	P	P

Name	Institution Internship/Residency	Fellowship Dates	Clinical Category	Research	Initial Career	Subsequent Career
Hines, James J.	Duke Medical Center	1981–84	G	B	A	P
Hinohara, Tomoaki	McGill University, Montreal, Canada	1982–85*	G–IC	C	A	P
Hlatky, Mark A.	U. Arizona	1981–83	G	C	A	A
Honan, Michael B.	Duke Medical Center	1986–89	G	C	P	P
Hurwitz, Jodie L.	Parkland—UTSW	1984–88	G–EP	B	A	A, P
Irwin, James M.	U. Pittsburgh	1985–88	G–EP	C	P	P
Jackman, J. Daniel	Parkland—UTSW—CR	1989–92	G–IC		P	P
Johnson, Eric E.	Bowman Gray	1989–94	G–EP	B	P	P
Jollis, James G.	Duke Medical Center	1989–92	G	C	A	A
Karas, Richard H.	Brigham & Women's Hosp.	1989–90*	G		A	A
Kay, G. Neal	U. Alabama, Birmingham—CR	1983–86	G–EP	C	A	A
Kitzman, Dalane W.	Mayo, Rochester	1987–90	G–REH	C	P	A
Kobilka, Brian K.	Barnes—Washington University	1984–89	G	B	A	A
Kort, Arthur A.	Indiana University Hosp. Albany Medical Center	1986–90	G	B	P	P
Krafchek, Jack	St. Vincent's Hosp., Australia	1983–85*	NIV	C	A	A
Kraus, William E.	Duke Medical Center	1986–88	G	B	A	A
Kryiakidis, Michael K.	U. Athens, Greece	1984–85*	G	C	A	A
Kuehl, William D.	The Ohio State Universtiy	1986–89*	G	B	A	P
Lee, Myoung M.	Seoul National University, Korea	1987–89*	IC	B	A	A
Leithe, Mark E.	The Ohio State University—CR	1987–89	G	C	P	P
Longabaugh, J. Peter	Duke Medical Center	1987–90*	G–NIV	B	A	P

Name	Institution Internship/Residency	Fellowship Dates	Clinical Category	Research	Initial Career	Subsequent Career
Lundergan, Conor F.	Duke Medical Center	1985–87 1988–89	G–IC	B	A	A, P
Manjoney, Dawn Y.	St. Vincent's Medical Center—Yale—CR	1989–90*	NIV		P	P, Ret
Mark, Daniel B.	U. Virginia, Charlottesville	1982–85	G	C	A	A
Martin, Jose C.	Jackson Memorial Hosp., Fl—CR	1982–84	G	C	A	P
McLeod, Andrew A.	United Kingdom	1981–83*	REH	C	A	P
Meese, Roderick B.	Parkland—UTSW	1985–87*	G–IV	C	P	P
Merrill, James J.	Parkland—UTSW	1989–93	G–EP	B	P	P
Miller, Michael J.	Duke Medical Center	1988–91*	G–EP	C	A	A, P
Moorman, J. Randall	Duke Medical Center—CR	1981–82 1983–85	G	B	A	A
Moreadith, Randall W.	Duke Medical Center	1986–88*	G	B	A	A, OMI
Morris, Pamela B.	Duke Medical Center	1984–86	G	B	A	P, A
Muhlestein, J. Brent	Duke Medical Center	1987–91	G–IC	B	A	A
Murray, Katherine T.	Vanderbilt	1985–87*	G–EP	B	A	A
Navetta, Frank I.	Duke Medical Center	1987–90	G–IC		P	P
Newman, William N.	Duke Medical Center	1981–83	G		P	P
O'Callaghan, William G.	Mast Misericordiae Hosp., Dublin, Ireland St. Vincent's Hosp., Dublin, Ireland	1983–86*	G–EP–IC	C	A	P
O'Connor, Christopher M.	Duke Medical Center—CR	1986–87 1988–89	G	C	A	A
Ohman, E. Magnus	St. Laurence's Hosp., Dublin, Ireland St. Vincent's Hosp., Dublin, Ireland	1987–91*	G–IC	C	A	A

Name	Institution Internship/Residency	Fellowship Dates	Clinical Category	Research	Initial Career	Subsequent Career
Packer, Douglas L.	Duke Medical Center	1983–85	G–EP	C	A	A
Page, Richard L.	Mass. General Hosp.	1987–89	G–EP	C	A	A
Parsons, William J.	Roger Williams Hosp., Brown University Strong Memorial Hosp., Rochester, NY	1985–88	G	B	A	P
Perez, Jose A.	Parkland—UTSW	1985–88	G–IC	B	A	P, A, P
Pierson, George B.	U. Kansas Medical Center—CR	1985–88	G	B	P	P
Poorbaugh, David M.	Mass. General Hosp.	1985	O		O	O
Quigley, Peter J.	St. Vincent's Hosp., Dublin, Ireland	1986–88*	IC	B	A	A
Radford, Martha J.	Brigham & Women's Hosp.	1981–84	G	B	A	A
Ramierz, Norman M.	Parkland—UTSW	1984–87	G–IC–EP		P	P
Roark, Steven F.	Duke Medical Center	1982–85	G	C	A	P
Robertson, Jeffery	Queen's University, Toronto, Canada	1983–84*	NIV	C	P	P
Sane, David C.	Duke Medical Center	1986–89	G	B	A	A
Schneider, Ricky M.	Mount Sinai, NYC	1980–83	G	B	A	P
Seaworth, John F.	Wilford Hall Medical Center, Lackland AFB	1980–82	G		OM	P
Shadoff, Neal	U. Colorado—CR	1982–84	G–IV	C	A	P
Sheikh, Khalid H.	U. Colorado—CR	1986–88	G	C	A	P
Shen, Win-Kugang	Mayo, Rochester	1986–88*	EP	B	A	A
Simonton, Charles A.	UCSF—CR	1984–86	G–IC	C	P	P, OMI
Sintetos, Anthony L.	Duke Medical Center	1983–87*	G	C	P	P
Skelton, Thomas N.	Parkland—UTSW	1984–87	G–IV	C	A	A

Name	Institution Internship/Residency	Fellowship Dates	Clinical Category	Research	Initial Career	Subsequent Career
Sketch, Michael H.	The Ohio State University	1987–90	G-IC	C	A	A
Smith, Ian D.	Strong Memorial Hosp., Rochester, NY	1981–83	G		P	P
Smith, Jack E.	U. Pittsburgh Hosp.	1987–90	G-IC		P	P
Smith, Mark S.	Johns Hopkins	1980–84	G-EP	B	A	P
Sorrentino, Robert A.	Duke Medical Center	1988–91	G-EP	C	A	A
Sprecher, Dennis L.	Michael Reese Hosp.	1985–86*	G	B	A	A, OMI
Sullivan, Martin J.	The Ohio State University	1984–86	G	C	A	A, P
Tang, Anthony S.	U. Ottawa, Canada—CR	1986–88*	EP	B	A	A
Tcheng, James E.	Barnes—Washington University	1986–89	G-IC	C	A	A
Teague, Stephen M.	Duke Medical Center	1980–83	G-NIV	C	A	P
Tenaglia, Alan N.	New York Hosp., NYC	1988–92	G-IC	B	A	P
Tomlinson, Charles W.	Hosp. Science Center, Winnepeg, Canada	1980–81*	NIV	C	A	A
Trahey, III, Thomas F.	Duke Medical Center	1987–89	G		P	P
Trantham, Joey L.	Duke Medical Center	1977–80	G-EP	B	P	P
Victor, Ronald G.	UCLA	1981–83*	G	B	A	A
Vidaillet, Humberto J.	Mayo, Rochester	1984–87	G-EP	B	P	P
Vitullo, Raymond N.	Mass. General Hosp.	1988–91	G-EP	C	P	P, Dec
Wall, Thomas C.	Duke Medical Center—CR	1985–86 1987–88*	G	C	A	P
Wefald, Franklin C.	Johns Hopkins	1987–90	G	B	P	P
Weiner, Henry L.	Temple University Hosp., Philadelphia	1986–90	G-EP	B	P	P
Wendt, David J.	Henry Ford Hosp., Detroit—CR	1989–92*	G-EP	B	A	P

Name	Institution Internship/Residency	Fellowship Dates	Clinical Category	Research	Initial Career	Subsequent Career
Wharton, J. Marcus	UCSF—CR	1984–87	G-EP	B	A	A
Wiseman, Alan H.	Royal Victoria Hosp., Montreal, Canada; Queen Elizabeth Hosp., Montreal, Canada—CR	1988–90*	G	B	P	P
Worley, Seth J.	Strong Memorial Hosp., Rochester	1981–84	G	B	A	P
Zidar, James P.	U. Michigan Medical Center—CR	1989–92	G-IC	B	A	A

See "Explanation for Data Tables" following Chapter II.

CHAPTER VI

1990–99

During the majority of the previous decade, I functioned as both Chief of Cardiology and Chairman of the Department of Medicine. Although this system undoubtedly had drawbacks, at least there was no haggling between Medicine and Cardiology regarding finances—a major positive feature. However, in 1989 for a variety of poorly thought out reasons, I made a decision to relinquish Cardiology. Accordingly, without benefit of a search process, Dr. Gary Stiles was named to lead the Division.

Gary continued to function as the Program Director. During the early part of the decade, both the recruitment strategies and the general curriculum remained essentially unchanged. For nearly all of the fellows, the Program was three years in duration: the time equally split between clinical and research training. The ability to construct a "tailor-made" program for each fellow remained feasible. However, a very significant decision by the American Board of Internal Medicine in 1987 began to gradually erode this option. Specifically, the board required that for the trainees to be eligible for board examination, the Program must be certified by the American Council on Graduate Medical Education (ACGME) (Chapter XII). At first, this rule seemed innocuous and reasonable. However, the wheels were set in motion so that curricula were less and less designed locally by the Program Director and the Chief of Cardiology; becoming dictated by a governing board of "self-appointed experts". As might be anticipated, the ACGME required extensive documentation as to the fellows' clinical activities, making the Program Director's job excessively tedious.

The first significant change was the requirement that the Program must contain at least two years of clinical cardiology which must be completed by the end of the third year of fellowship. Thus, the option to allow the trainee to carry out a two-year research experience at the beginning of the fellowship became very difficult to achieve. Although by no means universally the case, it has been advantageous for the fellow to be enmeshed in research training as soon as possible. Certainly, finishing several research projects in the initial years of the fellowship allowed the continuation of research during their clinical training, at least to some extent. This approach usually resulted in completed and published projects by the end of the fellowship. As far as basic research is concerned, a fellow without prior research experience is unlikely to choose a career in laboratory investigation if the individual has completed house staff and clinical cardiology training before beginning their basic research endeavor.

In 1994, Dr. Tom Bashore replaced Gary Stiles as Program Director and immediately increased the duration of the Training Program to four years. Linda Scherich assumed the responsibility for the administrative aspects of the Training Program. The number of fellows recruited each year was reduced by approximately 25 percent so that the total number of fellows remained unchanged. In order to preserve as much of the prior Program as possible, the design provided for an initial year followed by two research years and a fourth clinical year. This pattern was followed for several years before being rejected by the ACGME. The ACGME ruled that the first three years had to include two years training in clinical cardiology. This requirement usually forced the fellow to carry out the two-year period of research at the end of fellowship. The recruiting process changed significantly: Fellows were no longer matched to work with a given research preceptor. Also, a specific research interest or background in research was not the major factor in the selection process. Fellows were chosen, by and large, based on their superior clinical skills and a stated desire to become involved in academic cardiology.

Whether or not changes in the recruiting process were responsible, by the end of the decade, a decided shift in the research interests of the fellows occurred: The proportion choosing clinical vs. basic research shifted dramatically in favor of the former. Dr. Rob Califf developed a widely recognized and outstanding clinical trials unit, and although Dr. David Pryor left, the outcomes group primarily headed by Dr. Dan Mark also grew in statue. These research activities were consolidated and the Duke Cardiovascular Research Institute (DCRI) came into being in 1996. The overwhelming majority of the fellows finished their clinical training and spent two years in the DCRI in one of these two units. The shift away from basic research was essentially complete by the end of the decade. In 1999, none of the fellows were involved in any of the nine active basic research laboratories in Cardiology (Chapter IX, Table 2).

Another important aspect of the research training was the nearly universal desire of the fellows to participate in didactic course work. Dr. Bill Wilkinson, Professor of Biostatistics and Bioinformatics, developed an outstanding two-year course entitled "Health Sciences in Clinical Research". Ten of the cardiology fellows completed this work and received a Master's degree. The majority of the other trainees audited at least a portion of the course work.

Early in the decade, the Saturday conferences were discontinued. A weekly Cardiology Grand Rounds was instituted by Dr. Tom Bashore. The format was designed to present a core curriculum during the first six months. The rest of the year was reserved for presentations by visiting physician-scientists and individual fellows. A second weekly conference was instituted dealing primarily with diagnostic and therapeutic approaches to patients. Once a month, basic science topics were presented at this conference. A third weekly conference entitled "graphics-plus" explored a number of the techniques used in evaluating patients with cardiovascular disease. The Wednesday night research meetings continued, but attendance was sparse, at best.

The milieu for clinical training continued to expand in a number of areas. The Interventional Program, under the purview of Dr. Mike Sketch, continued to provide outstanding approaches to treatment. The separate match for interventional fellows was discontinued and training for intervention techniques was offered to all interested fellows. Thus, it was not necessary to go elsewhere for interventional training. This training took place during the time set aside for research and significantly altered the mix between dedicated research and clinical endeavors.

The Cardiac Catheterization Laboratory facilities were completely refurbished and consolidated on the seventh floor.

An "accommodation" was reached with Radiology so that a combined effort in peripheral vascular techniques was formulated. Led initially by Dr. Joe Perez and throughout the decade by Dr. Richard Stack, this Program involved the uses of intravascular procedures in the major arteries, including the carotids. A number of fellows from other institutions also participated in this Program.

One of the most durable and notable features of the Training Program continued through this decade: Drs. Vic Behar and Jess Peter precepting fellows in the techniques used in diagnostic cardiac catheterization. Their long-term commitment is truly a remarkable record. Both brought a mixture of outstanding expertise and good humor to this endeavor. Admittedly, Vic, who over the years was somewhat less patient with a slow learning fellow, frequently used his patented "hip shove" to nudge the fellow out of the way so that he could complete the task at hand. Famous for his whimsical comments, he delighted in noting that "without fellows, this would be a part-time job". When a fellow was floundering, he would often take a microphone and announce from the control room in the cath lab: "Please place the catheter down and slowly move away from the table". Then, he would burst into the lab and complete the study.

Jess was a character and much loved by the staff. He had an aversion to the morbidly obese and was often blunt in his comments. Vic delighted in switching cases so that Jess had to deal with such patients. One patient formally complained when Jess noted that her waist was so large "he could ski off her belly". To another, he once suggested that the patient was so fat that he had his own gravitational field!

In 1995, Dr. Tom Ryan was recruited from Indiana University to head the Cardiac Diagnostic Unit. He continued in the footsteps of Drs. Joe Kisslo and Bob Waugh by providing an outstanding clinical service and developed a number of research projects. Several of the fellows chose to carry out their research experience in this environment.

Dr. Marcus Wharton, continuing as the Director of Electrophysiology, developed an innovative approach to the intracardiac ablation of atrial flutter and fibrillation. A number of the fellows worked with Marcus to develop their ablation skills and in so doing, carried out clinical research. During this decade, there was a dramatic increase in the use of implantable devices, specifically pacemakers and defibrillators

Following the retirements of Drs. Bob Whalen and Bill Floyd, the Cardiovascular Disease Service became defunct. The general clinical load was assumed primarily by the physicians in the CAD Service which now included a number of cardiologists whose primary function was to carry out research in the DCRI. Thus, they had only a part-time role in clinical care. In addition, Dr. Tom Bashore, along with Dr. Kevin Harrison and later Drs. Andrew Wang, Gail Peterson, John Warner and Tom Gehrig, developed a clinical service, DHP (Duke Heart Physicians). The primary focus of this group involved the care of patients with adult congenital and valvular heart diseases and facilitated their clinical research program that focused on catheter interventions in these patients.

The total number of patients seen by these services gradually increased, with a very heavy emphasis on outpatient care. The outpatient facilities in Duke South were renovated. However, a number of cardiologists elected to follow their patients in the facilities at the Center for Living.

The Cardiac Rehabilitation Program continued primarily through the efforts of Drs. Fred Cobb and Bill Kraus.

This decade can be characterized as highly successful in restructuring the Program to a four-year commitment, recruiting outstanding physicians and providing superior clinical training. The emphasis on research switched nearly entirely to clinical investigation, primarily in the DCRI.

The Cardiology Fellows Training Program continued to have an excellent national reputation and attracted an increasing number of applicants.

Table 1 Cardiology Fellows: 1990–99

Name	Institution Internship/Residency	Fellowship Dates	Clinical Category	Research	Initial Career	Subsequent Career
Al-Khatib, Sana M.	Duke Medical Center	1996–00	G–EP	C	A	A
Alexander, John H.P.	Brigham & Women's Hosp.	1996–00	G	C	A	A
Alexander, Karen P.	Brigham & Women's Hosp.	1995–98	G	C	A	A
Ament, Alan S.	Duke Medical Center	1994–99	G	B	P	P
Amsterdam, Peter B.	Brigham & Women's Hosp.	1993–97	G–IC	C	P	P
Anderson, R. David	U. Maryland—CR	1994–98	G–IC	C	P	P, A
Armstrong, Brian A.	Duke Medical Center	1991–95	G–IC	B	P	P, OMI
Assar, Manish D.	Parkland—UTSW	1997–01*	G–EP	B	P	P
Bacon, Martin E.	Portsmouth Naval Hosp.	1990–91*	EP	C	A	P
Bahit, M. Cecilia	Hosp. Italiano de Buenos Aires, Argentina	1999–01*	NIV	C	A	A
Baker, William A.	UCSF	1993–96*	G–IC	C	A	A
Barold, Helen S.	Johns Hopkins	1994–98	G–EP	B	P	P, A, OMI, P
Barsness, Gregory W.	Duke Medical Center	1994–98	G–IC	C	A	A
Bart, Bradley A.	U. Colorado	1994–97*	G–NIV	C	A	A
Batchelor, Wayne B.	U. Toronto, Canada	1996–99*	G–IC	C	A	A, P
Battle, Judy K.	U. Alabama Hosp.	1996–00	G–EP	C	A	A, P, Dec
Biddle, William P.	Methodist Hosp., Memphis	1991–92*	IC		A	A
Blazing, Michael A.	UCSF	1991–95	G	B	A	A
Boineau, Robin E.	Miriam Hosp.—Brown University	1993–96	G	C	A	A
Boley, Jerry J.	Johns Hopkins	1993–96	G–NIV	C	P	P

Name	Institution Internship/Residency	Fellowship Dates	Clinical Category	Research	Initial Career	Subsequent Career
Botti, Jr., Charles F.	Wright-Patterson AFB Medical Center—CR	1993–94*	IC		OM	P
Brezinski, Damian A.	Beth Israel Hosp.	1992–94	G–IC	C	P	P
Brott, Brigitta C.	Beth Israel Hosp.	1991–95	G–IC	C	A	P, A
Cabell, Christopher H.	Duke Medical Center—CR	1997–98 1999–02	G–NIV	C	A	A, OMI
Callihan, Jr., Richard L.	Duke Medical Center	1992–95	G	B	P	P, A, P
Campbell, Kevin R.	U. Virginia, Charlottesville	1999–03	G–EP		P	P
Cantor, Warren J.	Toronto Hosp., Canada St. Michael's Hosp., Canada—CR	1998–00*	IC	C	A	A
Cohen, Mauricio G.	Hosp. Italiano de Buenos Aires, Argentina	1997–99*	IC	C	P	P, A
Cooper, Randolph A.S.	Duke Medical Center	1990–94	G–EP	B	A	A, P
Crenshaw, Brian S.	Duke Medical Center	1993–96	G	C	A	P
Cross, Jr., Andrew M.	East Virginia School of Medicine, Norfolk	1990–93*	G	C	A	A, P, A, P
Crow, J. Allen	Vanderbilt	1990–94	G	B	P	P, A
Crowley, James J.	U. Hosp., Galway, Ireland	1995–97*	IC	C	A	A
Cuffe, Michael S.	Duke Medical Center—CR	1994–95 1996–98	G	C	A	A
DeNofrio, David	Barnes—Washington University	1991–94	G	B	A	A
de la Serna, Fernando A.	Berkshire Medical Center, Pittsfield, MA	1998–00* 2003–07	G–IC	C	P	P
Dodds, III, G. Alfred	Medical College of Ohio	1992–95*	G–NIV	C	A	P
Donahue, Mark P.	U. Cincinnati	1999–03	G	B	A	A

Name	Institution Internship/Residency	Fellowship Dates	Clinical Category	Research	Initial Career	Subsequent Career
Drazner, Mark H.	Parkland—UTSW—CR	1993–96*	G	B	A	A
Dyke, Christopher K.	Parkland—UTSW	1998–04*	G–NIV	C	A	A, P
East, Mark A.	Duke Medical Center	1998–03	G–IC	C	P	P
Fanning, Thomas S.	The Ohio State University	1999–00*	IC		P	P
Federici, Robert E.	Stanford	1992–95	G–IC	C	P	P
Felker, G. Michael	Johns Hopkins—CR	1999–02*	G	C	A	A
Fennell, Maureen E. Collins	U. Maryland	1994–97	G–NIV	C	P	P
Forbess, Lisa W.	Mass. General Hosp.	1994–99	G–PED	C	P	P, A
Forrest, Terry L.	Duke Medical Center	1990–93	G	B	A	P
Fox, Jonathan C.	Duke Medical Center	1990–93	G	B	A	OMI
Freedman, Neil J.	Beth Israel Hosp.	1990–93	G	B	A	A
Gallagher, Peter L.	Parkland—UTSW	1997–01	G–EP	C	P	P
Gbadebo, T. David	Case Western Reserve	1997–99*	G		P	P
Gehrig, Thomas R.	U. Virginia, Charlottesville—CR	1998–02	G–IC	C	A	A
Greenbaum, Adam B.	U. Michigan	1995–99	G–IV	C	A	A
Gresham, Tina C.	Duke Medical Center	1990–93	G	C	P	P
Gruver, Carol L.	U. Connecticut	1991–94*	G	B	P	P
Hamer, Mark E.	Strong Memorial Hosp., Rochester, NY—CR	1990–94	G–EP	C	P	P
Hardee, Michael S.	Emory—Grady	1995–98	G–IC	C	P	P
Harrington, Robert A.	U. Massachusetts—CR	1990–93	G–IC	C	A	A

Name	Institution Internship/Residency	Fellowship Dates	Clinical Category	Research	Initial Career	Subsequent Career
Hathaway, William R.	Duke Medical Center—CR	1991–92 1993–95	G	C	P	P
Hearne, Steven E.	U. Maryland	1992–96	G–IC	C	P	P
Hesselson, Aaron B.	Beth Israel Hosp.	1997–01	G–EP	C	P	P
Hillegass, Jr., William B.	Brigham & Women's Hosp.	1991–95	G–IC	C	A	P, A
Hillsley, Russell E.	Duke Medical Center	1991–95	G–EP	B	P	P
Hochrein, James (Jake)	Duke Medical Center—CR	1993–95 1996–97	G–IC	C	A	P
Hsieh, Allen	Johns Hopkins	1994–97	G–NIV	C	P	P
Hudson, Michael P.	U. Michigan Medical Center—CR	1996–00	G	C	A	A
Javaid, Aamir	Duke Medical Center	1996–98	G		P	P
Kandzari, David E.	Johns Hopkins	1998–02	G–IC	C	A	A, OMI, A
Kao, Andrew C.	U. Minnesota	1991–95*	G	C	A	A, P
Kay, Joseph D.	U. Michigan Medical Center—CR	1999–04	G–PED	C	A	A
Kelsey, Anita M.	U. Connecticut—CR	1995–98	G–NIV	C	P	P
Kong, David F.	Johns Hopkins	1996–01	G–IC	C	A	A
Kong, Watakki	U. Toronto, Canada	1998–99*	IC		A	A
Kontos, Christopher D.	MCV, Richmond—CR	1993–97	G	B	A	A
Krasuski, Richard A.	Brigham & Women's Hosp.	1997–01	G–IC	C	OM (A)	OM (A), A
Kruse, Kevin R.	Duke Medical Center	1992–96	G–IC	B	P	P
Labinaz, Marino	U. Western Ontario, Canada—CR / U. Ottawa Heart Institute, Canada	1992–94*	IC	C	A	A
Lederman, Robert J.	Case Western Reserve—CR	1997–98*	IC	C	A	A

Name	Institution Internship/Residency	Fellowship Dates	Clinical Category	Research	Initial Career	Subsequent Career
Liao, Lawrence	Vanderbilt	1999–03	G	C	A	A
Lieberman, Eric B.	Johns Hopkins	1990–93	G-IC	C	OMI	P
Lim, Chang S.	U. Pennsylvania	1995–98	G-NIV	C	A	P
Madan, Minakshi (Mina)	Jewish General Hosp., McGill University, Canada; U. Ottawa, Canada—CR	1996–99*	IC	C	A	A
Mahaffey, Kenneth W.	U. Arizona Health Sciences Center—CR	1993–96	G-NIV	C	A	A
Martin, David O.	Beth Israel Hosp.	1996–00	G-EP	C	A	A
Mast, Steven T.	Johns Hopkins—CR	1997–01	G	C	P	P
Mayes, Jr., Charles E.	Parkland—UTSW—CR	1999–03	G-IC	C	P	P
McGuire, Darren K.	Parkland—UTSW	1997–01	G	C	A	A
McMullan, Michael R.	U. Mississippi Medical Center—CR	1997–98*	IC	C	A	A, P
Mendelsohn, Farrell O.	Mass. General Hosp.	1995–99	G-IC	C	P	P
Miller, Julie M.	Duke Medical Center	1995–99	G-IC	C	A	A
Morris, Edward I.	Duke Medical Center	1994–97	G-NIV	C	P	P
Nair, Lawrence A.	Johns Hopkins	1992–96	G-EP	B	P	P
Nathan, Paul E.	Jersey City Medical Center, NJ; St. Vincent's Hosp., NYC	1992*	G		P	P
Newby, Keith H.	Emory—Grady	1993–97	G-EP	C	P	P
Newby, L. Kristin	Duke Medical Center	1990–93	G	B	A	A
Nibley, Carleton T.	Oregon Health Sciences University	1992–95*	G-EP	C	P	P
O'Shea, J. Conor	U. Hosp., Cork, Ireland; Duke Medical Center	1998–02*	G	C	A	A

Name	Institution Internship/Residency	Fellowship Dates	Clinical Category	Research	Initial Career	Subsequent Career
Payne, Paul A.	Baylor, Houston, TX	1991–95	G	B	P	P
Petersen, II, John L.	Duke Medical Center—CR	1998–99 2000–04	G–IC	C	A	A, P
Peterson, Eric D.	Brigham & Women's Hosp.	1992–95	G	C	A	A
Peterson, Gail E.	Parkland—UTSW—CR	1995–99	G–NIV	C	A	A
Povsic, Thomas J.	Duke Medical Center	1998–04	G–IC	B	A	A
Pulsipher, Mark W.	Stanford	1993–97	G–IC	C	A	A, P
Rao, Sunil V.	Duke Medical Center	1999–04	G–IC	C	A	A
Rebeiz, Abdallah G.	Duke Medical Center	1999–03	G–IC	C	A	A
Richards, Adrienne L. •	Duke Medical Center	1995–97	G	B	P	P
Rigolin, Vera H.	Northwestern—CR	1992–95	G–NIV	C	A	A
Riley, Reed D.	Johns Hopkins	1991–95	G–EP	C	A	A
Robiolio, Paul A.	Brigham & Women's Hosp.	1992–95	G–IC	C	A	A, P
Russell, Stuart D.	Johns Hopkins	1994–97*	G	C	A	A
Safian, Robert D.	UCSD—CR	1997*	IC		A	A
Sanders, Jr., William E. (Gene)	U. North Carolina	1991–92*	EP	C	A	A, OMI
Santos, Renato M.	Duke Medical Center	1993–97	G–IC	B	P	P, A
Schnee, Janet M.	Mass. General Hosp.	1994–95*	G	B	A	A, OMI
Shah, Akbar	SUNY, Buffalo	1993–95*	G	C	A	P
Shah, Monica R.	Johns Hopkins	1997–02*	G	C	A	A
Shander, Gregg S.	U. Chicago	1994–98*	G–EP	C	P	P
Shenasa, Hossein	Sinai Samaritan, U. Wisconsin	1990–94*	G–EP	C	P	P

Name	Institution Internship/Residency	Fellowship Dates	Clinical Category	Research	Initial Career	Subsequent Career
Simons, Grant R.	Brigham & Women's Hosp.	1993–97	G–EP	C	P	P
Smith, IV, William T.	Mass. General Hosp.	1999–03	G–NIV–EP	C	P	P
Tan, Huay-Cheem	National U. Singapore	1995–96*	IC		A	A
Tan, June	Case Western Reserve	1998–99*	NIV	C	A	A
Tan, Melvin E. H.	Singapore	1995–96*	IC		P	P
Tanguay, Jean-Francois	Sacre-Coeur Hosp., Montreal, Canada / St. Luce Hosp., Montreal, Canada	1993–95*	IC	B	A	A
Thel, Mark C.	Portsmouth Naval Hosp. / Duke Medical Center—CR	1992–93 / 1995–97	G–IC	C	OM	P
Tice, IV, Frank D.	The Ohio State University—CR	1991–94	G–NIV	C	A	P
Tolleson, Thaddeus R.	Parkland—UTSW	1997–02	G–IC	C	P	P
Tomassoni, Gery F.	U. Hosp. Cleveland—CR	1994–98	G–EP	C	A	P
Tung, Chen Y.	Duke Medical Center	1995–99	G	C	P	P
Unks, Dennis M. (Mike)	Duke Medical Center	1990–93	G	C	OM	P
Velazquez, Eric J.	Duke Medical Center	1997–01	G	C	A	A
Vergara, Ismael A. •	Catholic University, Santiago, Chile	1997–98*	EP	C	A	A
Wang, Andrew	Johns Hopkins—CR	1993–94 / 1995–97	G–IC	C	A	A
Warner, John J.	Parkland—UTSW—CR	1996–00	G–IC	C	A	A
Whalley, David W. •	Australia	1992–94*	EP	B	P	P
Wharton, III, William W.	Letterman Army Medical Center, CA	1995–98	G	C	P	P
Whellan, David J.	U. Pennsylvania	1997–02	G	C	A	A
Whitehill, Jeffrey N.	Parkland—UTSW	1999–03	G–EP	C	P	P

Name	Institution Internship/Residency	Fellowship Dates	Clinical Category	Research	Initial Career	Subsequent Career
Wilson, John S.	Boston University—CR	1990–94	G-IC	C	P	P
Zabel, K. Michael	Duke Medical Center—CR	1991–92 1993–95	G	C	P	P
Zimerman, Leandro I.	Federal University Rio Grande, Brazil	1993–95*	EP	C	A	A

See "Explanation for Data Tables" following Chapter II.

CHAPTER VII

2000–09

The new millennium ushered in a series of events which would result in frequent changes in the leadership of Cardiology. Dr. Gary Stiles moved to an administrative position within the Duke Health System as Chief Medical Officer. During the search for a new Division Chief, Dr. Tom Ryan served as interim Chief of Cardiology.

For the first time in naming new leadership, an extensive national search was undertaken, spearheaded in large measure through Dean Sandy Williams' office rather than the Department of Medicine. Since Dr. Orgain's tenure, all of the Chiefs of Cardiology had been trained at Duke. The appointment of Dr. Pascal Goldschmidt ended this precedent. He had carried out research at Johns Hopkins and recently functioned as Chief of Cardiology at The Ohio State University. Dr. Tom Ryan retained the role as Clinical Chief of the Division as well as Director of the Heart Center. Dr. Tom Bashore continued as the Program Director.

Upon assuming command, Pascal initiated a number of strategies to augment the basic research functions of the Division. Shortly after he arrived, the training grant renewal was due. Although successful, a very significant problem noted by the review committee was that the number of cardiology fellows training in basic research had dwindled dramatically. Pascal committed his efforts to re-establishing the historical split, of fifty–fifty, between clinical and basic research training

Another goal which Pascal pursued was the development of Magnetic Resonance Imaging (MRI) facilities within Cardiology to be used both for clinical investigation and to augment patient care. Dr. Ray Kim was recruited from Northwestern to head this program. A number of fellows have elected to receive training and carry out clinical research utilizing this new technology.

The opportunity for the fellows to participate in basic investigation of interventional modalities was diminished when Dr. Richard Stack left the institution to pursue a career in industry. He made available the opportunity for fellows to be involved in research with him, and two fellows chose this pathway. However, unquestionably the closing of Richard's laboratory facilities significantly reduced the number of fellows who undertook research in invasive technology. In addition, with Richard's departure, interest in developing procedures to treat peripheral vascular disease waned.

In 2002, Dr. Marcus Wharton left to become Chief of Electrophysiology at the Medical University of South Carolina. After a year without a Director, Dr. Rob Sorrentino assumed this role. Dr. Rosie Gilliam, who had been practicing electrophysiology in Richmond, Virginia since finishing his fellowship, was recruited by Pascal in 2004 as the Director of Electrophysiology. In 2005, Rob Sorrentino left to become Chief of Electrophysiology at the University of Georgia Medical School in Augusta, Georgia.

After three years, Rosie returned to private practice. For two years, the Electrophysiology Service existed without a designated leader. Dr. Pat Hranitzky, a junior faculty member, was asked to shoulder the administrative load in the interim. In 2009, Dr. Jim Daubert was recruited to head the Electrophysiology Service. Jim completed both his house staff and cardiology fellowship training at Duke and also was a Chief Resident in Medicine. He has been extremely productive as Chief of Electrophysiology at the New York University at Rochester, New York. Currently, he is in the process of re-organizing the Electrophysiology Service and recruiting additional physicians. New updated EP laboratories were completed in 2009 and a major expansion of the EP facilities is expected by 2012.

In July 2003, Pascal became Chairman of the Department of Medicine. Following a national search, he appointed Dr. Pam Douglas, an echocardiographer who was Cardiology Chief at the University of Wisconsin, to become Chief of the Division of Cardiology. (In April 2006, Pascal left to become Dean at the University of Miami.) Tom Ryan continued as the Director of the Heart Center and as the Clinical Chief of the Division until his departure to The Ohio State University in 2006.

During her first year as Division Chief (2004), Dr. Pam Douglas functioned as President of the American College of Cardiology. For a variety of reasons, she relinquished her role as Chief of the Division in 2006. In the spring of 2007, Dean Sandy Williams appointed Dr. Howard Rockman as Chief of Cardiology. Dr. Chris O'Connor became Director of the Heart Center. Tom Bashore assumed the generally thankless role as Clinical Director of the Division. Thus, the administrative functions of the Division were jointly assumed by the triumvirate of Drs. Rockman, O'Connor and Bashore. Sherolyn Patterson ably carried out the administrative functions of the Training Program.

In order to expand the patient service area, the leadership of DUMC made a decision to purchase the Raleigh Community Hospital and changed the name to Duke Raleigh Hospital. The facilities for cardiovascular patients were less than optimal, making it difficult to compete with both Wake and Rex Hospitals. In spite of these limitations, Dr. Jim Zidar, who accepted the responsibility, developed a strong cardiology program, especially in the treatment of patients with peripheral vascular disease. Cardiology fellows participated in this program. The Divisional leadership decided to support the development of a Heart Center in Lumberton. This activity not only required considerable effort by several of the senior cardiologists in the Division, but also resulted in a significant reduction in patient referrals from this area. Fellow participation was limited to a lucrative moonlighting opportunity. The Duke Health System also purchased the Durham Regional Hospital but did not change the name.

In 2005, Dr. Svati Shah became the Assistant Training Program Director. Among her other duties, she assumed the role of organizing the weekly Cardiology Grand Rounds. The material presented at this conference, both clinical and research, has, in general, been outstanding. Although well attended by the fellows, attendance by the senior Cardiology faculty has been sparse.

The role of overseeing and mentoring the Training Program remained on Tom Bashore's capable shoulders until 2008 when Dr. Andrew Wang became the Program Director.

The size of the Training Program remained essentially static during the decade. Eight four-year fellows are chosen each year along with an unspecified number who obtain training for one – two years in the various subspecialties.

In order to recognize the contributions of Dr. Jess Peter to the Interventional Program, a fellowship in Interventional Cardiology was begun in 1999. The awardees were chosen based on their clinical expertise in interventional cardiology. The following were named the Jess Peter Interventional Cardiology Fellow:

1999	Thaddeus R. Tolleson
2000	Charles E. Mayes, Jr.
2001	David E. Kandzari
2002	John L. Petersen, II
2003	Sunil V. Rao
2004	Frederick J. Meine, III
2005	Kanwar P. Singh
2006	Richard P. Konstance, II
2007	George L. Adams
2008	Daniel R. Guerra
2009	W. Schuyler Jones

All good things come to an end sooner or later! In 2006, both Drs. Jess Peter and Vic Behar officially retired—leaving a very difficult gap to fill in cardiac catheterization training.

In 2007, Dr. Kevin Harrison replaced Dr. Mike Sketch as Director of the Cardiac Catheterization Laboratory. In the same year, Dr. Eric Velazquez became Director of the Cardiac Diagnostic Unit (CDU). Dr. Chris Granger remained as Director of the CCU. Dr. Ken Morris continued to function as the Chief of Cardiology at the Durham Veterans Affairs Medical Center. These venues provide the bulk of training in diagnostic procedures.

The DCRI continued to be the primary outlet for training in clinical investigation within the Cardiology Division. As in the previous decade, a number of the fellows have chosen to participate in a two-year clinical research training program leading to a Master's degree.

The long-standing Wednesday night research meeting was canceled. The clinical cardiology training conferences, noted in the previous decade, were augmented. Another "Core Cardiology" conference has been initiated which deals with a number of topics including ECG reading sessions, practice guidelines, as well as basic science reviews. If the number of didactic conferences defines success in cardiology training, the current group of fellows should be the best ever.

In order to provide a similar opportunity for fellows interested in basic or translational research, a Master's program in Genomics was initiated in 2004. The opportunity to carry out basic research in laboratories within the Division was reduced when Dr. Goldschmidt left and Dr. Brian Annex became Chief of Cardiology at the University of Virginia in Charlottesville. Dr. Geoffrey Pitt was recently recruited in basic electrophysiology and has developed a productive laboratory. The approach during the decade to increase the number of cardiology fellows electing to become involved in basic research has been reasonably successful. In the current academic year (2009) 38 percent of the fellows who are involved in research training are in basic investigation. (Chapter IX, Table 2). Unfortunately, the majority are studying in non-cardiology research laboratories. A major win for basic research was scored when Dr. Matt Wolf, working with Howard Rockman, won the coveted American Heart Association Katz Prize for Young Investigators at the 2005 annual meeting. As in the previous decade, the majority of the fellows who carried out clinical research do so with one of the investigators in the DCRI.

Because of significant pressure from the accrediting agencies, the strategy to have the fellows complete their clinical training prior to a significant research experience now is firmly established, with only an occasional exception to this rule. Thus, the opportunity to individualize the fellowship to meet the interest of the given fellows has been significantly reduced.

The Cardiology Division has continued to provide an adequate volume of patient care activities which are essential for the clinical training of fellows. In 2009, 3,373 diagnostic catheterizations and 944 interventional procedures were performed. In addition, there were 605 coronary artery bypass operations. The volume of these procedures was about 75 percent of those carried out in 1990.

The bulk of the patients cared for by Cardiology either are through the CAD (Cardiology at Duke) or the DHP (Duke Heart Physicians) Services. The Heart Failure Service, headed by Dr. Chris O'Connor, has expanded considerably. The cardiac transplant program received a major boost when Dr. Carmelo Milano became the surgical director and Dr. Joe Rogers, recruited from Barnes, the medical director.

The primary Duke cardiology outpatient facilities moved from Duke Hospital South and the Center for Living to a large clinical space in both northern Durham (North Duke Street) and in southern Durham (Southpoint). These clinics significantly enhance the ability of the Cardiology Division to deliver care in easily accessible locations and to train fellows.

Table 1 Cardiology Fellows: 2000–09

Name	Institution Internship/Residency	Fellowship Dates	Clinical Category	Research	Initial Career	Subsequent Career
Abraham, Dennis M.	Mount Sinai, NYC—CR	2007–p	G	B		
Adams, George L.	Parkland—UTSW	2003–07	G–IC	C	A	A
Adams, Joseph C.	U. Mississippi Medical Center	2002–03*	IC		P	P
Albert, Timothy S.E.	U. Washington	2002–06	G–NIV	C	P	P
Allen, Larry A.	Mass. General Hosp.	2004–07	G–NIV	C	A	A
Ambati, Srivani R.	Allegheny University Graduate Hosp.	2004–05*	NIV		P	P
Amos, Ankie-Marie	Duke Medical Center	2003–06	G–NIV	C	A	P
Anderson, Monique L.	Vanderbilt	2009–p	G			
Ang, Gregory B.	Johns Hopkins	2003–07	G–NIV	C	P	P
Atchley, Jr., Allen E.	Duke Medical Center	2006–p	G–NIV	C		
Atwater, Bret D.	Duke Medical Center	2008–p*	EP	C		
Bensimhon, Daniel R.	Duke Medical Center	2001–05	G–REH	C	A	P
Berger, Jeffrey S.	Beth Israel—CR	2005–08*	G	C	A	
Berman, Adam E.	Georgetown	2004–06*	EP	C	A	A
Biswas, Mimi S.	Cedars-Sinai Medical Center	2001–04	G	C	A	P
Bloomfield, Jr., Gerald S.	Johns Hopkins	2007–p	G	C		
Brennan, J. Matthew	U. Chicago	2006–p	G	C		
Brosnan, Rhoda B.	Parkland—UTSW—CR	2001–05	G–NIV	C	P	P
Campbell, Mark E.	Keesler AFB Medical Center	2002–03*	IC		OM	OM, P
Choi, Kelly M.	Northwestern	2002–04*	G	C	OMI	OMI
Contrafatto, Igino	U. Bologna, Italy	2003–04*	EP	C	A	A

Name	Institution Internship/Residency	Fellowship Dates	Clinical Category	Research	Initial Career	Subsequent Career
Crowley, Anna Lisa Chamis	Duke Medical Center	2001–05	G-NIV	C	A	A
Dellock, Carey D. Moyer	Penn State—CR	2005–06*	IC		P	P
Dery, Jean-Pierre	Laval University, Canada	2001–03*	IC	C	A	A
Diamantouros, Pantelis	McMasters University, Canada U. Western Ontario, Canada	2006–07*	IC	C	A	A
Dixon, IV, William C.	Brooke Army Medical Center—CR	2001–02*	IC	C	OM	OM, P
Durrani, Sarfraz, A.K.	Georgetown—CR	2004–06*	EP		P	P
Eapen, Zubin J.	Duke Medical Center	2008–p	G	B		
Echols, Melvin R.	Duke Medical Center—CR	2007–p*	G	C		
Egnaczyk, Gregory F.	Mass. General Hosp.	2006–p	G	B		
Farzaneh-Far, Afshin	Brigham & Women's Hosp.	2007–09*	NIV	C	A	
Fischi, Michael C.	SUNY, Syracuse	2000–04*	G	B	P	P
Fortin, Terry Ann	Duke Medical Center	2002–06	G	C	A	A
Frazier-Mills, Camille G.	Duke Medical Center—CR	2002–03 2004–09	G-EP	C	A	
Gharacholou, S. Michael	Duke Medical Center	2005–09*	G-NIV	C	A	
Goswami, Robi	Duke Medical Center	2009–p	G			
Goyal, Abhinva	U. Pennsylvania	2002–07	G	C	A	A
Guerra, Daniel R.	Brigham & Women's Hosp.	2004–09	G-IC	C	P	
Hainer, Mark I.	U. Hawaii—CR	2006–07*	IC		OM	OM
Haithcock, Daniel B.	Temple—CR	2004–08	G-EP	C	A	P
Halabi, Abdul R.	McGill University, Montreal, Canada	2003–05*	IC	C	P	P

Name	Institution Internship/Residency	Fellowship Dates	Clinical Category	Research	Initial Career	Subsequent Career
Halim, Sharif	Duke Medical Center	2009–p	G			
Harrison, Robert W.	Duke Medical Center—CR	2008–09	G	B		
Hegland, Donald D.	Duke Medical Center—CR	2003–07	G–EP	C	A	A
Heitner, John F.	Duke Medical Center	2002–04*	NIV	C	A	A
Hernandez, Adrian F.	UCSF	2000–04	G	C	A	A
Hess, Connie Ng	Mass General Hosp.	2009–p	G			
Hess, Paul L.	Mass. General Hosp.	2009–p	G			
Hranitzky, Patrick M.	Parkland—UTSW	2000–04	G–EP	C	A	A
Jackson, Kevin P.	UCSF	2003–07	G–EP	C	A	A
Javaheri, Sean P.	Tripler Army Medical Center	2008–09*	IC		OM	
Jolicoeur, E. Marc	Montreal University, Canada	2008–09*	IC		A	
Jones, W. Schuyler	Duke Medical Center—CR	2004–05 2006–p	G–IC	B,C		
Karra, Ravi	Brigham & Women's Hosp.	2008–p	G	B		
Katz, Jason N.	Parkland—UTSW—CR	2005–09	G	C	A	
Kaul, Prashant	Presbyterian Hosp., NYC	2006–p	G–IC	C		
Khouri, Michel G.	Parkland—UTSW—CR	2008–p	G			
Kiefer, Todd L.	Stanford	2007–p	G–IC	C		
Kindsvater, Steven M.	Keesler AFB Medical Center	2003–04*	IC		OM	OM
Kinney, Kurt G.	Tripler Army Medical Center	2005–06*	IC		OM	OM, P
Kociol, Robb D.	Brigham & Women's Hosp.	2007–p	G	C		
Kong, Melissa Huang Szu-Min	Duke Medical Center	2007–p	G–EP	C		

Name	Institution Internship/Residency	Fellowship Dates	Clinical Category	Research	Initial Career	Subsequent Career
Konstance, II, Richard P.	Duke Medical Center	2002–07	G-IC	C	P	P
Koontz, Jason I.	Duke Medical Center	2004–p	G-EP	B		
Kransdorf, Evan P.	Duke Medical Center	2009–p	G			
Kunz, Geoffrey A.	Duke Medical Center—CR	2000–01 2002–05	G-IC	C	P	P
Lam, Gregory K.W.	Duke Medical Center	2004–09	G	B	P	
Lim, Ing Haan	Singapore General Hosp.	2005–06*	IC		P	P
MacKay, Steven M.	Lutheran General Hosp., Park Ridge, IL	2009–p*	IC			
Markham, David W.	U. Virginia, Charlottesville	2002–04*	G	B	A	A
Mehta, Rajendra H.	J.J. Groups of Hospitals, University of Bombay, India Catholic Medical Center, Cornell University	2003–04*	IC	C	P	P
Meine, III, Frederick H. (Tripp)	Duke Medical Center	2001–05	G-IC	C	P	P
Mills, James S.	Brigham & Women's Hosp.	2003–08	G-IC	B	A	A
Mitchell, Robert G.	UCSF	2002–06	G	B	A	A, P
Mudrick, Daniel W.	Brigham & Women's Hosp.	2007–p	G-NIV	C		
Mulhearn, IV, Thomas J.	Johns Hopkins	2007–p	G-IC	B		
Nilsson, Jr., Kent R.	Johns Hopkins	2005–p	G-EP	B		
Nguyen, Can Manh	McGill University, Montreal, Canada	2000–02*	IC	C	A	A
Patel, Chetan B.	Parkland—UTSW—CR	2006–p	G	B		
Patel, Mahesh J.	Parkland—UTSW	2007–p	G	C		
Patel, Manesh R.	Duke Medical Center—CR	2000–01 2002–06	G-IC	C	A	A

Name	Institution Internship/Residency	Fellowship Dates	Clinical Category	Research	Initial Career	Subsequent Career
Perzanowski, Christian A.	Loma Linda University	2004–06*	EP		P	P
Piccini, Sr., Jonathan P.	Johns Hopkins	2005–p	G–EP	C		
Rajagopal, Sudarshan	Duke Medical Center	2008–p	G	B		
Russo, Cheryl A.	Duke Medical Center	2001–05	G–NIV	C	P	P
Salerno, Michael	Stanford	2005–08	G–NIV	C	A	A
Samad, Zainab	Duke Medical Center	2005–09	G–NIV	C	A	
Sastry, Ashwani	Presbyterian Hosp., NYC	2009–p	G			
Schwender, Frank T.	Henry Ford Hosp.	2005–07*	EP		P	P
Senthikumar, Annamalai (Senthil)	Advocate IL Masonic Medical Center, Chicago	2007–09	NIV		A	
Seo, David M.	Beth Israel	2000–04	G	B	A	A
Shah, Bimal R.	Stanford	2005–09	G	C	A	
Shah, Svati H.	Brigham & Women's Hosp.	2001–05	G	C	A	A
Singh, Kanwar P.	Brigham & Women's Hosp.	2002–06	G–IC	C	A	A
Stavens, Gerasimos S.	St. Louis University Hosp.	2001–02*	EP		P	P
Stiber, Jonathan A.	Duke Medical Center	2000–04	G	B	A	A
Subherwal, Sumeet	Barnes— Washington University	2008–p	G			
Sun, Albert Y.	Duke Medical Center—CR	2006–07 2008–p	G–EP	B		
Thomas, Kevin L.	Duke Medical Center—CR	2002–03 2004–07	G–EP	C	A	A
Trichon, Benjamin H.	Johns Hopkins	2000–04	G	C	P	P
Trimble, Mark A.	U. Michigan Medical Center	2004–08	G–NIV	C	P	P

Name	Institution Internship/Residency	Fellowship Dates	Clinical Category	Research	Initial Career	Subsequent Career
Turer, Aslan T.	Duke Medical Center	2004–09	G-IC	C	A	A
Valente, Anne Marie	Duke Medical Center	2001–06	G-PED	C	A	A
Van de Car, David A.	Brooke Army Medical Center	2009–p*	IC		A	
Vavalle, John P.	U. North Carolina—CR	2008–p	G			
Vemulapalli, Sreekanth	UCSF—CR	2009–p	G			
Voora, Deepak	Barnes—Washington University	2006–p	G	C		
Wallace, Thomas W.	Parkland—UTSW—CR	2006–p	G-EP	C		
Wang, Tracy Y.P.	Brigham & Women's Hosp.	2004–07	G	C	A	A
Ward, Cary C.	Parkland—UTSW	2002–07	G	B	A	A
Waters, Richard (Rip) E.	Johns Hopkins	2001–05	G-IC	B	P	P
Williams, Eric S.	UCSF—CR	2008–p	G			
Wince, William B. (Ben)	Emory—Grady	2008–p*	NIV	C		
Wolf, Matthew J.	Duke Medical Center	2003–07	G	B	A	A
Yager, Jonathan E. E.	UCSF	2001–05	G	C	P	P
Zidar, David A.	Johns Hopkins	2001–p	G-IC	B		
Zidar, Frank J.	U. Michigan Medical Center—CR	2004–05*	IC		P	P

See "Explanation for Data Tables" following Chapter II.

CHAPTER VIII

RECRUITMENT

As would be anticipated during the first two decades of the Program, the majority of the fellows (73 percent and 67 percent, respectively) did, at least, some of their house staff training at Duke (Table 1). Several others trained with Dr. Stead or his colleagues when they were at Emory. Thus, the recruitment was essentially "in house" and consisted entirely of individual agreements made during the latter part of house staff training.

In the third decade, the Program became better known both within the United States as well as internationally. The stated goals to train academic cardiologists made the Program attractive to a growing number of house staff interested in pursuing a career as an academic cardiologist. In addition, during the initial period, a significant number of the graduates of the Program who had gone to other academic institutions recommended the Program to the house staff. One of the strong influences regarding the international reputation came from development of basic and clinical electrophysiology: fellows came to Duke specifically to train in this subspecialty. During the last four decades, the percentage of fellows who, at least, had some house staff training at Duke, decreased and became relatively constant, 23–31 percent (Table 1).

Recruitment from geographic sections of the country in the six time periods revealed several interesting trends. During the first two time periods, excluding the Duke trainees, approximately nine percent were from the Northeast, eight percent from the Southeast and eight percent from the Midwest. From 1970 through 2010, the decrease in trainees from Duke was offset by a significant increase from other sections of the country. During the last four time periods, each section of the country was represented. Recruitment from the Northeast ranged from 18 to 30 percent; Southeast, five to ten percent; Southwest, six to nine percent; Midwest, ten to 20 percent and Far West, four to ten percent. During the past two time periods, the significant increase in the Northeast to 30 percent was due in large measure to recruitment either from Johns Hopkins or Brigham and Women's Hospital. These two institutions accounted for 38 percent of the fellows recruited from the Northeast. The fellows recruited from the Southwest came almost exclusively from UTSW.

By the early 1970s, there were significantly more applicants than available positions. A more formal interview process, including a mandatory on-site interview, was initiated. Although there were significant exceptions, the majority of the fellows were accepted into the Program during their training as a junior assistant resident. This early acceptance was dictated, to a large measure, by significant changes in funding sources. As noted in Chapter X, the initial training grants provided by the NHI were designated to train clinical cardiologists. These funding sources ceased and training money became available only for research training. Initially, these were individual grants requiring the description of a specific research project. Thus, the prospective fellow had to be chosen so that there was enough time available for submitting a grant prior to the beginning of the fellowship. Since the philosophy of the Program had shifted to having the majority of the fellows carrying out significant research, the earlier acceptance date became mandatory. When institutional training grants became available in the mid 70s, the concept of early acceptance was not altered.

The number of fellows accepted each year gradually increased to a steady state of 12–15 during the 80s and 90s. When the duration of training was increased to four years, the number entering the Program yearly was reduced to 8–10.

Table 2 documents the percentage of cardiology fellows who had functioned as a Chief Resident in Internal Medicine during their training. During the last two decades, this group has increased to 24 and 22 percent, respectively

During the late 70s, formal interview days were initiated wherein the prospective trainee visited the institution. They were evaluated by a number of the faculty including a faculty member who might serve as the individual's mentor. When the interviews were completed, the applicants were ranked and then notified in the May–June time frame, i.e., approximately 13 to 14 months prior to their beginning date. The selection was related primarily to matching a fellow's interests with a specific research mentor. The field of research chosen was frequently unrelated to a subspecialty in cardiology, although it was generally assumed that individuals interested in basic research in electrophysiology would more than likely become electrophysiologists. Similarly, research interest in hemodynamics would be expected to lead to a subspecialty career in cardiac catheterization procedures.

Since many of the top ranked fellows were recruited by other training programs, friction began to develop nationally. The recruiting process became more intense and significant pressure was put on the fellows to accept positions prior to the time they learned whether they could go elsewhere. This was never a serious problem at Duke, but in many other programs, recruitment policy was considered to be a significant national issue. So much so, that during the mid 80s, a Cardiology Match Program "reared its ugly head". Conceptually, this procedure worked in a manner similar to the house staff matching program. However, at least at Duke, the match created significant problems; it became very difficult to be certain that research fellows could be recruited to the positions available in the various research laboratories. For this reason, during the initial two to three years of the match, Duke "opted out". When we did become involved, only a portion of the fellows recruited were actually put into the match. As with any Program of this type, significant chicanery developed. A number of program directors, although espousing loyalty to the concept of a match, continued to put pressure on the fellows for early commitment. Frankly, at a time in which the problems related to cheating in cardiovascular research was being given a lot of press, "bending" the match rules as their initial exposure to the Program certainly sent the wrong message to the prospective fellow.

By the early 90s, the general concept of matching fellows to specific research laboratories essentially disappeared. This enabled complying with the rules of the match much easier. During the last decade, the match has been strictly adhered to and the fellows chosen through this mechanism. For the past two decades, the fellows have been accepted based on their potential to be outstanding cardiologists. Most of them expressed an interest in research, generally, clinical. During the past five years, a concerted effort has been made to recruit fellows interested in basic research.

Throughout the last three decades, the number of applicants interested in cardiology training at Duke has soared. For the past several years, more than three hundred applications have been received for each of the available positions.

As the reputation of the Training Program spread, a number of foreign trained physicians applied (Table 3). For the period 1970–1999, 13 percent of the trainees were foreign. Most of these had prior cardiology experience and came for specific training opportunities, e.g., electrophysiology, interventional cardiology or cardiovascular research. In general, these physicians were outstanding. For the current decade, seven percent of the trainees were foreign.

The number of women and black physicians entering the Training Program is provided in Table 4. The significant increase in the number of female physicians choosing cardiology during the past two decades mirrors the increase in the number of women entering medical school. However, the choice of cardiology as a medical subspecialty, at least in the Training Program at Duke, has been significantly less among females as compared to male physicians.

During the past decade, a concerted effort has been made to recruit black physicians into the Training Program. The results have been moderately successful—seven percent in the current decade.

Table 1 Recruitment from the Duke House Staff

1946–59	1960–69	1970–79	1980–89	1990–99	2000–09
73%	67%	31%	28%	23%	28%

The percent of cardiology fellows receiving at least some of their training in Internal Medicine at Duke.

Table 2 Recruitment of Chief Residents

1946–59	1960–69	1970–79	1980–89	1990–99	2000–09
17%	12%	10%	17%	24%	22%

The percent of cardiology fellows who had been a Chief Resident in Internal Medicine.

Table 3 Recruitment of Foreign Physicians

1946–59	1960–69	1970–79	1980–89	1990–99	2000–09
7%	5%	15%	12%	12%	7%

Percent of cardiology fellows who received house staff and/or cardiology training at a foreign institution.

Table 4 Recruitment of Blacks and Women

1946–59	1960–69	1970–79	1980–89	1990–99	2000–09
0%	1%	3%	2%	4%	7%
0%	0%	4%	10%	13%	16%

The percent of black physicians recruited into the Program is listed in the first row.
The percent of female physicians recruited into the Program is listed in row two.
Six percent of the female physicians are black.

CHAPTER IX

CURRICULA

The salient features of the structure of the Training Program for both the clinical and research components are outlined for each decade in Chapters II – VII. The purpose of this chapter is to give a broad overview highlighting the evolution of the Training Program.

In a nutshell, the Program can be characterized initially as a *laissez-faire* approach, i.e., learning opportunities from the patients and preceptors were available, but it was entirely up to the individual to educate himself. The schedules for the Cardiovascular Disease Service fellows under Dr. Orgain dictated specific clinical duties. Schedules for the fellows under the Stead group were essentially nonexistent. It was entirely possible for a fellow to skip a major area of cardiology, e.g., cardiac catheterization, and still complete requirements for the Cardiovascular Disease Board examination. Research training was entirely under the aegis of the preceptor and, in general, the trainees learned how to do research by doing research.

As the procedures related to cardiovascular disease become more complex, schedules were gradually altered so that the fellows, as a general rule, had an opportunity to learn these modalities. The dramatic growth of echocardiography in the 70s is a case in point.

Throughout the 60s and early 70s, the general format of the Program required that a fellow be assigned primarily to one preceptor for his clinical training. For example, fellows worked with either Dr. Orgain or Dr. McIntosh and the majority of the training was obtained in their venues. During the latter part of the 60s, this concept began to break down so that fellows started rotating for specific periods through the various clinical components, i.e., CCU, Cardiovascular Disease Service, Cardiac Catheterization Laboratory or the DVAH.

In the 1980s, the philosophy changed so that an 18-month core curriculum was instituted containing all aspects of cardiology. Additional clinical training could be obtained in interventional cardiology or electrophysiology. However, the general program was structured so that 18-month clinical training was coupled with an 18-month period of research. During the period 1960–89, approximately one-half of the fellows carried out basic and one-half, clinical research. However, during the past two decades, clinical research has predominated (Table 1). Recently, an increasing number of fellows have opted to train in basic research—40 percent in 2009 (Table 2).

It is interesting to examine the changing scene regarding various procedures. Although electrocardiography has remained an important key technique throughout the entire training period, it has obviously assumed a less dominant role. Vector-cardiography, as both an important clinical entity and as a mechanism for teaching electrocardiography, played a role in the 70s and 80s but due to the unreimbursable costs, it has essentially disappeared. Continuous ECG monitoring for arrhythmias was ushered in with the advent of the CCU. This approach has been expanded to the non-acute patient by using the techniques of Holter or loop monitoring. Phono-cardiography, which was widely employed both as a diagnostic tool and to teach physical diagnosis, has disappeared. Ballistocardiography briefly saw the "light of day" in the early 60s but the clinical utility of this technique did not prove to be worthwhile.

The development of echocardiography had a major impact on the Training Program and a number of the fellows chose this subspecialty as a major component of their clin-ical and research training. Nuclear cardiology also made a major impact on the eval-uation of patients with cardiovascular disease. Housed in the Department of Radiol-ogy as a training modality, it has not assumed the deserved premiere role in Cardiology. During the past decade, MRI facilities within Cardiology have allowed the fostering of a robust clinical and research program.

Perhaps no other aspect of cardiology had a more dramatic growth than cardiac catheterization. Initially employed for hemodynamic assessment using right heart catheterization, it has evolved to include definitive interventional approaches for in-travascular atherosclerotic disease in both cardiac and peripheral vessels. The growth in interventional cardiology, as well as electrophysiology, spawned the development of subspecialty boards in both of these entities. Thus, additional training is necessary to be board eligible.

In the past decade, the training has been expanded to a full two-year commitment in clinical cardiology. Standard rotations are taken by each fellow, covering every as-pect of cardiology. Subspecialization in either electrophysiology or interventional car-diology requires additional clinical training. Also, in order to have a "marketable" skill, many of the fellows have elected to receive additional training in noninvasive technol-ogy. Unfortunately, these clinical commitments invariably decrease the time available for research. Thus, for many of the fellows, dedicated research training plays "second fiddle" in the current curricula.

Another distinct change in the clinical Training Program has been the significant increase in the number of didactic conferences—currently four/week. For people who learn by attending conferences, the current format should be ideal.

The nature of research training has been altered considerably in that the over-whelming majority of fellows are not involved in basic research but are carrying out clinical investigation primarily at the DCRI. Formal course work in a variety of clini-cal research techniques has been undertaken; a number of the fellows have completed the two-year Master's course entitled "Health Sciences in Clinical Research".

In a nutshell, it is clear that the nature of the Training Program and the curricula have evolved from a generally *laissez-faire* approach, which allowed the fellows to "pick and chose", what they wanted to master. In fact, they might omit formal training in a given discipline. The fellows were responsible for their own training structure. Now the Program has a much more stereotype approach in which every fellow must com-plete a fairly comprehensive core curriculum. Similarly, the research training has evolved from primarily on the job "learning to do research by doing research" to en-compassing a significant component of didactic course work.

Mentoring, obviously an important aspect of the Training Program, is performed at different levels. To be effective, mentoring must include not only scientific direction but also fostering the development of a long-term research goal.

Initially, the primary mentor was the director of the area in which the fellow elected to work. After Dr. McIntosh assumed the role as Chief of the overall Division, he initiated the concept that the Division Chief should function as an important mentor. With the advent of a Program Director, separate from the Division Chief, this individual became a key part of the mentoring effort. This process has continued until the present. The second level of mentoring has been provided by the leader of the research laboratory in which the fellow participated. Undoubtedly, this aspect of the Program has been an important feature of its success. (The influence of a specific mentor on the choice of an academic career is detailed in Chapter XIII.)

Although he was officially in charge of the Training Program for only five years, Dr. Galen Wagner played a major role in mentoring the fellows in clinical research. During a 40-year period, 86 fellows authored or co-authored either peer-reviewed manuscripts or book chapters with Galen. Seventy-six of these published manuscripts during their fellowship and 34 continued to publish additional papers with Galen after the fellowship. The number of papers per fellow ranged from one to sixteen. It is obvious from these data that Galen had a major impact on the publication productivity of a number of fellows.

Table 1 Research Training

1946–59	1960–69	1970–79	1980–89	1990–99	2000–09
43%	53%	63%	89%	92%	77%
15%	60%	49%	52%	22%	18%
85%	40%	51%	48%	78%	82%

Row 1 lists the percentage of fellows finishing the Program who received specific research training in their fellowship.

Rows 2 and 3 list the percentage of fellows trained in either basic or clinical research, respectively.

The period 1990–99 can be divided further. Physicians entering the Program before 1995: 34% and 66% received basic or clinical training, respectively.

Physicians entering the Program after 1995: 8% and 92% received basic or clinical training, respectively.

Table 2 Training Assignments at End of Each Decade

	1969	1979	1989	1999	2009
Total	16	30	51	39	41
Clinical Rotations	12	15	30	23	23
Research Rotations	4	15	21	16	18
Basic Research	4	8	13	0	7
Clinical Research	0	7	8	16	11
Basic Laboratories	3	8	13	9	10
Clinical Laboratories*	1	6	7	6	9

Row 1 lists the total number of fellows in the Program for the specific year indicated in the columns.

Rows 2–5 list the number of fellows assigned to a particular Program.

Rows 6–7 list the basic and clinical laboratories available, respectively.

Only basic laboratories are listed in which the laboratory director's primary appointment is in the Cardiology Division. An asterisk indicates that the DCRI was counted as two laboratories (clinical trials and outcomes).

CHAPTER X

FUNDING

This chapter contains two aspects of funding: 1) fellow salaries during their training and 2) research activities of the fellows during their career.

When the fellowships started, the stipend ($2400/year) was obtained primarily from Dr. Orgain's professional fees. Shortly after his arrival in 1947, Dr. Stead was contacted by the leadership of the National Heart Institute (NHI) and informed him that they would like to provide a stipend to the Department of Medicine to train a cardiology fellow. Dr. Stead's response was "No, but if you'll send two stipends per year, I'll take them." After a brief pause, this format was agreed upon and the formal NHI supported training grant became a reality. (The process now is somewhat more involved!)

Dr. Stead made available one of these stipends to Dr. Orgain, giving a stable funding mechanism for at least one of the fellows each year. In 1959, an NHI Training Grant was awarded (HE05369) and in 1965 a second training grant (HE05736) was funded. Unfortunately, precise information as to the number of fellows supported by these grants cannot be ascertained. The philosophy of these grants was to train clinical cardiologists with the primary goal that a significant number would pursue a career in academic medicine.

It is somewhat unclear when these training grants were officially phased out but by 1970, they were no longer available. The NHI took the position of supporting only that component of the training which was specifically research oriented. This decision added to the already significant problem of obtaining funds to support fellows.

Individual, but not institutional, grants to support research training were available prior to 1975. In order to have the grant funded at the time the fellowship began, the grant had to be submitted at least a year prior to the time the training grant was activated. As described previously, this dramatically altered the recruitment process and the fellows had to be identified in time to prepare a submission for funding.

In 1975, an institutional training grant in cardiovascular research was awarded with Dr. Andy Wallace as the principal investigator. Although other clinical departments were involved, the majority of the stipends were used to support cardiology trainees, but only during specific research activities. This grant is currently active and directed by Dr. Howard Rockman (HL007101-35). The number of stipends varied from a high of 15 to the current level of eight. In 2003, a Clinical Research Training Grant (HL69749) supporting three stipends was awarded by the National Heart, Lung & Blood Institute. Dr. Dan Mark is the principal investigator.

Throughout the entire existence of this Training Program, as one might expect, fellows who were able to obtain their own funding were given preference. Dr. Barry Ramo's experience highlighted this situation. Barry had trained at the University of Chicago in Internal Medicine and applied for fellowship at Duke. However, he was given little encouragement. After successfully obtaining a research training grant award, he was welcomed into the Program—money always prevails.

Although there are other reasons for the significant increase in the number of foreign trained physicians in the Program during the 1970s, the fact that they arrived fully funded undoubtedly added to the interest in their participation.

As a general rule, the research mentor was responsible for salary funds for the fellow. In addition to NHI research fellowships, there were a number of NHI research grants in which stipends for fellows were available. For example, the Myocardial Infarction Research Unit (MIRU) grant supported fellows carrying out research in patients with acute myocardial infarction. A variety of other sources were utilized to support the research training of the fellows.

During the past century, there was a constant scramble to obtain funds to support fellows during their clinical training. A number of sources were utilized. Money from the professional charges of the senior cardiologists was designated to support fellows during their clinical rotations. The DVAH from its inception (1953) allocated funds for house staff and fellow training. Two to four stipends per year were derived from this source. Fellow support from DUMC was allocated from specific clinical entities, e.g., the Cardiac Care Unit, Cardiac Catheterization, Electrophysiology Laboratories and the Cardiac Diagnostic Unit. Finally, the outreach program provided an important salary source.

During the past decade, funding the clinical training has become less haphazard. Currently, DUMC and DVAH (three salaries) provide money for the basic stipends for the fellows during their clinical rotations. However, depending on the grade level, these may have to be supplemented to some extent.

Endowments have not been a significant source of fellow support, with one exception: The Walter L. Floyd Endowed Cardiology Fellowship. In 1993, a cardiology fellowship was named for Bill. Fellows chosen were judged to be among the best clinicians. The appointment as a Floyd Fellow is highly prized. The following fellows received this award:

1993	K. Michael Zabel	2002	Benjamin H. Trichon
1994	Eric D. Peterson	2003	Rhoda B. Brosnan
1995	Jerry J. Boley	2004	Terry A. Fortin
1996	Andrew Wang	2005	Larry A. Allen
1997	Gail E. Peterson	2006	Jonathan P. Piccini, Sr.
1998	John J. Warner		
1999	Manish D. Assar	2007	Chetan B. Patel
2000	Thomas R. Gehrig	2008	Todd L. Kiefer
2001	William T. Smith, IV	2009	John P. Vavalle

Dr. Floyd clearly was an outstanding clinical cardiologist, but more importantly, he was a role model who exhibited the finest attributes of a physician. Rounding with Bill was considered to be one of the top experiences by the fellows during their clinical rotations. Bill also made a major commitment to the teaching of medical ethics, especially during the latter part of his career.

The following estimates research funding obtained by the fellows from the National Institutes of Health, the American Heart Association, the Veterans Administration, and industries. The data for the fellows remaining at Duke during their academic career is reasonably complete. However, for the fellows at other academic institutions, it is quite likely that a significant number of funding sources were not identified. Thus, the data undoubtedly significantly underestimate the total research funding.

For the purposes of this presentation, research and training grants awarded to the fellows by the National Institute of Health (NIH) were characterized as follows: Individual Research (R01, R03, R09, R29, R37), Program Research (P50, P60, P41), Contracts (N01, N43, N44), General Research Centers (M01), Institutional Training (T01, T15, T32, T35), Career Development Award (K03, K04, K08) and Miscellaneous which includes Cooperative Agreements (U09, U76), and Shared Instrumentation/Equipment (507, 515). In order to be included, the fellow had to be the principal investigator of an individual grant or of a project within either a program or a center grant. Regardless of the duration of the grant or multiple primary investigators, a given grant or project is listed only once. Grants categorized as defined above are listed in Table 1. The duration of the grant is given as up to five years, five to ten years, or greater than ten years.

From examining Table 1, it is obvious that the fellows pursuing academic careers were extremely successful in obtaining funding from a variety of different mechanisms through the NIH.

The American Heart Association provided significant support for the cardiology fellows. During the period from 1948–present, nine individuals received an Established Investigator Award. There were 70 research and 11 miscellaneous awards.

A number of fellows received research funding through the Department of Veterans Affairs. Throughout the period, there were 17 specific research grants or Merit Reviews and 13 either Research Associate or Clinical Investigator Awards. In addition, fellows were extremely successful in obtaining individual research grants from industrial sources.

Contracts with industry were extremely important in funding the research activities of the fellows. For example, industrial grants supported the research endeavors of the Cardiology Interventional Laboratory. In addition to research support, a large number of equipment donations were obtained including x-ray, echocardiographic, electrocardiographic, and other laboratory equipment.

Although the precise amount of financial support from all of these sources is unavailable, it should be clear that the fellows were remarkably successful in obtaining research support through a variety of peer review and non-peer review sources.

In 1995, I stepped down as Chairman of the Department of Medicine. The Joseph C. Greenfield, Jr. Scholars Program was initiated in my honor. These funds were designed to be used to support the research activities of young investigators. In 2001, the Greenfield Scholar in Cardiology Program was started. Yearly, an individual in Cardiology receives a $25,000 stipend to support their research. To date, ten individuals have been named as Greenfield Scholars in Cardiology. Their names and current academic affiliations are listed in Table 2.

Table 1 NIH Funding

	0–5 Years	5–10 Years	> 10 Years
Individual Research	96	57	20
Program Research	28	24	8
Contracts	7	6	3
General Research Centers	13	3	9
Institutional Training	8	4	3
Career Development Award	16	2	
Miscellaneous	7		

The categories listed in each row in column one were based on prefix designations as defined in the text. The total number of awards of specific duration are listed in columns 2–4.

Table 2 Greenfield Scholars in Cardiology

Date	Name	Current Position
2001–02	Eric J. Velazquez	Director, Cardiac Diagnostic Unit Associate Professor of Medicine, DUMC
2002–03	Christopher H. Cabell	Sr. Director, Medical and Scientific Services Quintiles, Durham, NC
2003–04	David J. Whellan	Associate Professor of Medicine Jefferson Medical College, Philadelphia, PA
2004–05	Svati H. Shah	Assistant Professor of Medicine, DUMC Assistant Director, Cardiology Fellows Training Program
2005–06	Manesh R. Patel	Assistant Professor of Medicine, DUMC
2006–07	Matthew J. Wolf	Assistant Professor of Medicine, DUMC
2007–08	James S. Mills	Assistant Professor of Medicine, DUMC
2008–09	Gregory K.W. Lam	Cardiology Practice, Columbus, OH
2009–10	Gerald S. Bloomfield	Cardiology Fellow, DUMC
2010–11	Jonathan P. Piccini, Sr.	Assistant Professor of Medicine, DUMC

The dates of appointment, the names, current affiliation and academic rank, if applicable, are listed in Columns 1, 2, and 3 respectively.

CHAPTER XI

OUTREACH

Following the mandate of James B. Duke regarding the purpose of the Medical Center component of Duke University, the Cardiology clinical service grew as a consequence of providing outstanding clinical care. The majority of the patients were referred by physicians within North Carolina. The first program within the Department of Medicine to attract patients on a national basis was Dr. Walter Kempner's rice diet therapy for the treatment of hypertension. The concept of providing clinical services at locations outside of DUMC by the senior cardiologists was infrequent. (Perhaps the best example of a Duke outreach program was developed within the Orthopaedic Service under the direction of Dr. Lenox Baker. Almost from its inception, the orthopaedic staff serviced a number of clinics scattered throughout North Carolina.)

In 1972, the impetus for developing outreach capability in Cardiology began with the development of the collaborative program at Cabarrus Memorial Hospital (renamed Northeast Medical Center—NMC) in Concord, NC. This venture between the physicians at DUMC and those at NMC developed under the tutelage of Dr. Stead and was supported in part by the Cannon Foundation. The primary purpose was educational, and so far as Cardiology was concerned, consisted of cardiology fellows spending four days per month per fellow at NMC. Two fellows at a time were assigned to this program. Their specific duties were to present teaching conferences, see patients in consultation for the medical staff and when indicated, facilitate the referral of patients to DUMC. Duke provided a Program Director for Internal Medicine, Dr. Galen Wagner, who spent two days per week coordinating the program—one day at NMC and one at DUMC.

The 120 mile each way weekly commute to NMC offered Galen the opportunity to try out his new sports car. Unfortunately, the speed limit, 55 mph, posed a problem. In fact, Galen soon accrued enough speeding tickets to result in either the loss of his driver's license or mandatory participation in extensive driver re-education. Galen opted to take to the air; for many years he utilized a local airplane service. In the past several years, with the advent of a higher speed limit and the development of a "lighter foot", Galen reinstituted the automobile commute.

The NMC Program was extraordinarily successful. In 1989, following his training in cardiology at DUMC, Dr. Tom Trahey became the Director of Cardiology at NMC. As the program expanded, two additional fellows (Drs. Paul Campbell and Kevin Kruse) joined the group. Over the next decade, other subspecialists in Medicine joined the staff at NMC; interest in learning from the "Duke fellows" waned. Consequently in 2000, the Fellow Program was replaced by senior staff consultation via interactive video conferences.

It is important to reiterate that the primary focus was educational for both the fellows and the physicians at NMC but did not function primarily as a mechanism for referral of patients to DUMC. The principle "carrot", as far as Cardiology was concerned, was the money derived from the program to pay the entire salary of two cardiology fellows.

A second, although minor area of outreach, was the VA Hospital in Fayetteville, NC. Both fellows and senior staff physicians consulted approximately once per month at this facility.

The impetus to expand the outreach program to other communities was fostered primarily by the funds from the North Carolina Area Health Education Program (AHEC). This program was developed exclusively to provide continuing medical education to physicians practicing in communities within North Carolina. Funds primarily supported patient care oriented lectures to the local physicians. Because of his expertise developed by running the program at NMC and his interest in outreach, Dr. Galen Wagner assumed the responsibility of coordinating these programs for the Department of Medicine. Rather than simply provide lectures, he used the NMC model to set up clinics where the fellows could see patients for the local physicians, and thus function as consulting cardiologists. Supervision was provided by local physicians, depending on the level of expertise, and also by the senior cardiologists at DUMC. As a general rule, the fellows enjoyed the outreach assignments because it gave them the opportunity to provide cardiology services to a very appreciative rural population. This successful concept was expanded dramatically and became an established part of the Training Program. By 1980, there were ten similar programs in existence. The success of this endeavor was primarily related to the efforts of Galen, ably assisted by Judy Berry.

Although not as financially lucrative to the Cardiology Division as the NMC program, these endeavors did provide significant funds to offset the fellow salaries. As the program expanded, most of the fellows were involved with one of the programs for at least a year of their fellowship.

Gradually, the emphasis began to shift from purely educational to providing a mechanism to facilitate the referral of patients to DUMC for cardiovascular consultation and work-up or direct admissions for acute care.

In order to provide echocardiographic facilities to a number of the outreach sites, an echo van was outfitted. Fellows participated in this venture. Several years later, a similar approach was developed to provide cardiac catheterization service by utilizing a mobile cath lab.

When the helicopter service became a reality in 1985, the primary function was not acute trauma, but the urgent care of patients with acute cardiovascular syndromes. In fact, for a number of years, more than 70 percent of the patients transferred via helicopter were admitted to the Cardiology service. The presence of the outreach program in a number of communities facilitated the ability of the helicopter transport service to become functional quite rapidly.

During the 1980s, the outreach program expanded dramatically. By the end of the decade, there were 18 communities serviced through this mechanism (Figure). As the program grew, additional staff was employed. Specifically, Tom Revels, who later became Hospital Director at NMC, was extremely helpful in developing the expanded outreach program. By and large, the format developed earlier continued to be employed; the cardiology fellows had a primary impact on the quality of the program.

By 1990, the outreach program had expanded into many areas of medicine. It became a hospital function initially under the direction of Jim Knight and later Malcolm Isley with three other full-time administrators. The outreach program began to be a very important mechanism for the referral of patients to DUMC. Data from the mid 90s indicated that, of the patients referred to Cardiology within North Carolina, 50–60 percent originated from communities in which a viable outreach program was in effect.

During the past decade, the magnitude of the outreach program for the cardiology fellows has been gradually decreased. The primary issue has not been one of available outreach locations but primarily dictated by potential legal issues. In this age in which concerns over medical malpractice have accelerated, issues regarding the appropriate coverage of the fellows while on outreach activities were judged to be a serious problem. The legal mavens ruled that it was mandatory that a senior cardiologist be present at the time the fellow was engaged in outreach activities. The logistics of this situation became essentially impossible to schedule. The bottom line is that the last outreach program for the cardiology fellows was closed in July 2009. Although to my knowledge, no malpractice situation related to inadequate senior staff coverage occurred during outreach activities, but this fact did not win the day. Unfortunately, the best interests of both patients and fellows did not prevail over the legal roadblocks. Outreach finis!

Although not specifically part of the training mission, moonlighting increased dramatically so that currently a very large percentage of the fellows moonlight. Although by no means a teaching function, moonlighting has provided the opportunity for the fellows to use their cardiology expertise, frequently referring patients to DUMC. During the 80s, moonlighting was officially frowned upon, and the fellows performed the service *sub rosa*. Several somewhat comical incidents occurred involving acutely ill patients arriving at DUMC having been referred by one of the moonlighting fellows. Since their moonlighting had not been officially sanctioned, considerable consternation was generated, especially by the DUMC legal staff.

Moonlighting became officially sanctioned in the mid 1990s and has continued to flourish. The amount of moonlighting which is currently allowed has been controlled via the mandated GME working hours. (Probably this is the only worthwhile result from the meddling of this august body.) Since only 80 hours of clinical activities per week is mandated, the fellows can moonlight only up to a total of 80 hours including their assignments in the Training Program. Since most of their assignments during the clinical rotations require at least 60 hours per week on site, the amount of moonlighting allowed is significantly curtailed. In fact, on a number of the clinical rotations, moonlighting simply cannot be carried out.

The fellows must notify the Training Program Director of all moonlighting activities. Depending on the nature of the activity, the malpractice insurance is covered either through DUMC i.e., Durham Casualty, or the administrative head of the moonlighting site. Fellows cannot moonlight unless it is judged that activities are adequately covered by malpractice insurance.

So moonlighting is here to stay. At least there is a mechanism for controlling the negative effects on the Training Program.

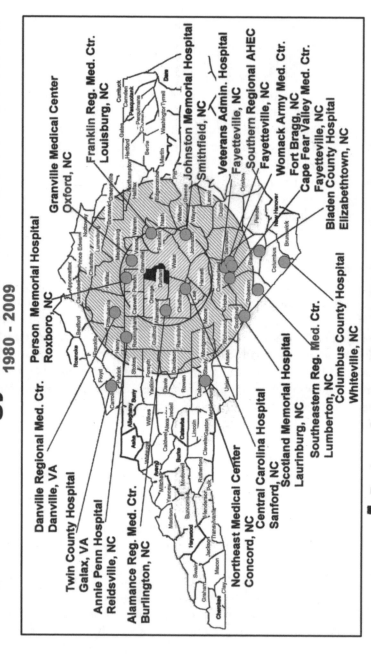

Duke Cardiology Fellow Outreach Clinics
1980 - 2009

Danville Regional Med. Ctr.
Danville, VA

Twin County Hospital
Galax, VA

Annie Penn Hospital
Reidsville, NC

Alamance Reg. Med. Ctr.
Burlington, NC

Northeast Medical Center
Concord, NC

Central Carolina Hospital
Sanford, NC

Scotland Memorial Hospital
Laurinburg, NC

Southeastern Reg. Med. Ctr.
Lumberton, NC

Columbus County Hospital
Whiteville, NC

Person Memorial Hospital
Roxboro, NC

Granville Medical Center
Oxford, NC

Franklin Reg. Med. Ctr.
Louisburg, NC

Johnston Memorial Hospital
Smithfield, NC

Veterans Admin. Hospital
Fayetteville, NC

Southern Regional AHEC
Fayetteville, NC

Womack Army Med. Ctr.
Fort Bragg, NC

Cape Fear Valley Med. Ctr.
Fayetteville, NC

Bladen County Hospital
Elizabethtown, NC

Durham County - Duke University Medical Center

Fellow Clinic

Up to 1-hour drive

1 - 2 hour drive

CHAPTER XII

CARDIOVASCULAR DISEASE BOARDS

Since one of the primary goals of the Fellowship Training Program was to prepare the trainee for the examination by the Subspecialty Board in Cardiovascular Disease, a brief review of the board requirements would seem to be in order.

The Subspecialty Board in Cardiovascular Disease was formed and the first examination administered in 1941. At that time, the credentials of each applicant were approved on an individual basis by the Cardiovascular Disease Advisory Board (CDAB). Initially, the criteria were not precisely defined. However, during the period from 1941 to 1970, the CDAB generally required at least one year of training in Cardiovascular Disease which was taken within the training period required for certification in Internal Medicine. The specific policy stated: "Four years of training in Internal Medicine and Cardiovascular Disease after the completion of an internship." Thus, the total training time was five years after graduation from medical school. Many of the internships at that time were rotating and did not count as specific training for Internal Medicine. Initially, it was possible to take three years of Internal Medicine training and one year of Cardiovascular Disease and still be eligible. After straight medical internships became acceptable as fulfilling the criteria for Internal Medicine Boards, most fellows trained in cardiovascular disease for a two-year period in order to complete the five-year training program. In addition to this training, a variable period of time practicing as a cardiovascular specialist was required. For example, between 1959–64, candidates were not eligible to apply for admission to the Cardiovascular Subspecialty Board until three years after certification in Internal Medicine. In 1965, this period was reduced to two years.

In 1970, the CDAB stipulated that a two-year period of training in the subspecialty was necessary.

It is of considerable interest that the Board did not define the contents of the training program but relied on the program director to certify that the applicant had received sufficient training in cardiovascular disease. This *laissez-faire* attitude was extremely important in allowing multiple different tracks to be employed.

In 1987, the CDAB changed the requirements so that the training must have been completed in a fellowship training program accredited by the ACGME. Thus, the contents of the training program shifted from the purview of the program director to a standardized format directed by a bureaucratic national committee.

Beginning in 1993, the Board required three years of accredited training containing a minimum of 24 months clinical training.

In the initial period of the fellowship 1946–59, certification by the Subspecialty Board in Cardiovascular Disease was not universally sought by the trainees, whereas certification in Internal Medicine was a high priority. In fact, Dr. Putt Pryor indicated that there was little interest in Cardiovascular Subspecialty Board certification among his colleagues.

The Table lists the percent of trainees certified by Internal Medicine and Cardiovascular Disease Boards. Whereas the overwhelming majority were certified in Internal Medicine throughout the entire period, during the initial years, a much smaller percent obtained certification in Cardiovascular Disease.

Subspecialty certification in electrophysiology and in interventional cardiology became a reality in 1992 and 1999, respectively. In order to be certified as eligible for examination by either of the subspecialty boards, detailed and rigorous training curricula were required.

Board Certification

1946–49	1960–69	1970–79	1980–89	1990–99	2000–09
28	60	95	132	132	68
86%	90%	95%	98%	99%	97%
43%	75%	92%	95%	98%	93%
	1	7	30	21	6
		7	28	37	16

The number of trainees eligible for board examination is listed in the first row.
The percent certified in Internal Medicine and Cardiovascular Disease is given in the second and third rows, respectively.
The fourth and fifth rows list the number (not percent) of fellows certified in Electrophysiology and Interventional Cardology, respectively.

CHAPTER XIII

CAREERS

From its institution through June 2009, a total of 564 fellows enrolled in this Program finished their training in cardiology. (Four additional fellows elected to pursue other careers.) Forty-one fellows currently are in training. In this chapter, the careers of these trainees in the years following the completion of their fellowship are summarized. The material is presented in two sections: 1) academic and 2) non-academic. When possible, the factors that entered into their career choices will be elucidated. Much of the pertinent source material is contained in the data tables at the end of Chapters II–VII.

Academic

For the period 1946 – 2009, 564 fellows completed training at Duke; 58 percent chose an initial academic career. As might be anticipated, a large number, 169, of these physicians began their career at DUMC. Of the 329 fellows who began an academic career, 226 or 69 percent have spent their predominant career in academia. (The predominant career was determined for each fellow who had finished the fellowship for at least a one-year period and was based on the higher percent of time spent in either an academic or non-academic career.) The predominant career of 72 of these physicians (32 percent) was spent at DUMC.

Tabulation of the initial career choice of the 74 recent graduates (Table 1) indicates that 58 percent were academic with 65 percent of these remaining at Duke. Of the 29 recent graduates having a predominant academic career, 55 percent remained at Duke. In comparison, only 29 percent in the years 1946–1999 had a long-term Duke career.

The percentage of fellows remaining in academia in the years following fellowship is illustrated in Figures 1–4.

Figure 1 depicts the percentage of 96 fellows finishing the program from 1946–69, who remained in academia each year during a follow-up period of 30 years. As might be anticipated, there is an abrupt decrease during the first five years among the Duke physicians. After a ten-year period, 39 percent of the group remained in academia. A slight decrease to 35 percent occurred after a 20-year follow-up and remained essentially constant thereafter. Twenty percent of the fellows began their academic career at another institution. During the follow-up period, this percentage actually increased to 25 percent due to the recruitment of cardiologists from DUMC by other academic programs.

Similar data are illustrated in Figures 2–4 for the periods 1970–79 (109 fellows), 1980–89 (144 fellows), and 1990–99 (141 fellows) respectively. The attrition rate is remarkably similar to that noted in Figure 1, for the 30-year (Figure 2), and the 20-year (Figure 3) follow-up periods. In contrast, there is only a minimal attrition rate for the

1990–99 ten-year follow-up period with a higher percentage remaining at Duke (Figure 4). The attrition rate for fellows beginning their career at Duke (1946–89) should be viewed from the following perspective. Many of the fellows who were undecided as to their future direction at the end of their fellowship remained at Duke an extra year or two as associates in Medicine in order to carry out research or to pursue additional clinical expertise. Then they decided to pursue a non-academic career. When the duration of the Training Program was increased to four years (1994), this option disappeared and is primarily responsible for the low initial attrition rate noted in Figure 4. Another responsible factor for the attrition rate is the number of fellows who transferred from Duke to another academic institution. During the 1946–2009 period, 33 fellows made this career choice with a high percentage, 76, occurring during the first five years of their academic career.

In comparing Figures 1–4, it is interesting to note that in the time periods illustrated, in Figures 1 and 3, a greater percent of the fellows began their academic career at Duke, whereas the reverse occurred in the time periods illustrated in Figures 2 and 4. The reason for this discrepancy is unclear. In examining the Figures, the long-term trend is clearly a decrease in the percentage remaining in academia; however, occasionally for a given follow-up year, this trend is reversed. Throughout the entire period illustrated in these four Figures, 29 (9.6 percent) individuals moved from a non-academic to an academic career — at least transiently. Eighteen of this group had chosen a non-academic initial career.

For the period 2000–09, a year-by-year follow-up was not plotted since the period of time is not adequate to make meaningful conclusions. It should be noted that the initial academic career choice of 58 percent of the fellows is in line with the previous decades. The shorter follow-up period in this group makes the 67 percent predominant career in academia difficult to compare with the preceding decades.

The career choices of 135 fellows trained at Duke from 1970–84 was reported by Pritchett et al.[1] A life table analysis was used to predict the attrition rate from academic careers. A linear seven percent per year reduction was estimated for a 10-year follow-up period. When compared to the actual data, the sharp drop off during the first five years was missed by the model. In addition, the model over estimated the actual per year attrition rate of five percent.

The administrative academic positions held by fellows are listed in Table 1. It is obvious that graduates of the Program have made a significant impact in this aspect of academic medicine. For the first five time periods, 22 percent of those remaining in an academic career served as Division Chiefs. The Chairmanship of 16 departments was held by the former fellows. In addition, for the first four time periods, 68 percent who had a long-term academic career were Professors and 33 percent of these became Distinguished Professors. In evaluating the administrative positions and the academic ranks of the fellows in the last two time periods, it should be remembered that the short follow-up period of time after finishing their fellowship precludes a reasonable assessment of their ultimate status.

Several fellows had top leadership roles in the national cardiology associations: Drs. Henry McIntosh and Doug Zipes served as President of the American College of Cardiology and Dr. Gus Grant was the President of the American Heart Association.

Are there any characteristics of the fellows which might be used to predict the choice of an academic vs. a non-academic career? For the entire group (564), 58 percent chose an initial academic career and of that group, 69 percent remained in academia. In Table 2, a number of characteristics that might have affected their choices are depicted.

It is apparent that the foreign fellows have a higher likelihood of remaining in academia. In fact, of the 65 foreign fellows, 77 percent embarked on an academic career. The reason for this seems obvious, since by and large they were chosen by their respective institutions to receive training at Duke and then return to an academic job.

The other characteristics examined namely, Chief Medical Resident, Duke House Staff and those who carried out either clinical or basic research—did not yield a subgrouping which was markedly different from the average (Table 2). For the entire period, 134 fellows did not have dedicated research training. In this group, only 35 percent elected academia as their initial career choice.

In order to further evaluate the personal aspects of the trainee which might have influenced their career choice, a detailed questionnaire (Appendix) was solicited. Significant debt at the end of fellowship training is often ascribed as a major cause of the choice to eschew an academic career. However, assuming the results of this survey are correct, none of the fellows finishing before 1969 had very significant debt, i.e., greater than $50,000 (related to dollar value in 1980). In the groups 1970–79, 1980–89, and 1990–99, 5 and 13 and 4 fellows, respectively, reported this level of debt. However, of these 22 fellows, 9 chose academia and 13 chose practice careers. Thus, the level of debt would not seem to have a major significant influence on their career undertaking. Whether or not the fellows were married also was not found to be pertinent. Similarly, a stated goal to pursue an academic career at the beginning of fellowship was not predictive. One characteristic seems to be significant: fellows choosing an initial academic career publish more during their training (Chapter XIV).

One final aspect of the training curricula on career choices was examined: How important was a specific mentor? The mentor of each fellow carrying out either clinical or basic research was identified. For mentors who were responsible for at least five fellows, the career choices of these fellows were characterized. Of the 22 mentors evaluated, fellows choosing an academic career ranged between 35 and 80 percent with Dr. Harold Strauss taking the top honors. Obviously, there was no way to determine the amount of time spent between a given mentor and a fellow or to precisely evaluate the other aspects of the relationship.

What is very clear from the foregoing: The fellows finishing the Cardiology Training Program at DUMC made a large impact on academic cardiology both in the United States and abroad. Unfortunately, comparative data from other training programs are not available. It would be surprising however, if the Duke record has been surpassed.

Non-Academic

For the period 1946–2009, the majority of the 330 fellows who pursued a predominately non-academic career chose the practice of cardiology. However, 17 fellows chose other endeavors—including careers in the military or the pharmaceutical industry.

The pertinent characteristics describing the nature of their practice are summarized in Table 3. As might be anticipated, the vast majority of fellows entered a group practice. Interestingly, a number of these group practices contained more than one cardiology fellow trained at Duke (ranging from 25–54 percent).

The nature of the individual practice is categorized. During the initial three periods, general cardiology, which includes imaging and diagnostic catheterization, was predominant. However, the advent of interventional treatment procedures e.g., angioplasty and electrophysiology, led to further subspecialization of the practices. For the last two decades, 60 percent of the fellows are primarily engaged in one of these two subspecialties. An impressive number of fellows participated in clinical trials.

As might be anticipated, a very high percentage of the fellows carried out administrative functions for the hospital in which they practiced. In addition, a number had an administrative role in their practice.

The overwhelming majority of the fellows are members of the American College of Cardiology and a number carried out administrative roles for their local American Heart Association or American College of Cardiology.

Table 3 lists the number of fellows with clinical appointments at an academic institution, indicating that a significant number played a role in either the teaching or research activities of these institutions.

From the above data, it is quite obvious that the Duke fellows in practice contributed significantly to health care related activities in their local medical communities.

Table 1 Career Summary—Academic

	1946–49			1960–69			1970–79			1980–89			1990–99			2000–09		
Graduates (Total)	30			66			109			144			141			74		
Academic Career																		
Initial	11	37%	(8–73%)	35	54%	(20–57%)	61	56%	(26–43%)	97	67%	(55–57%)	82	58%	(32–37%)	43	58%	(28–65%)
Predominant	10	91%	(3–30%)	26	72%	(8–31%)	38	64%	(7–18%)	59	61%	(15–25%)	65	81%	(23–35%)	29	67%	(16–55%)
Administrative Positions																		
Dean/Associate Dean	0			2/1			1/7			0/1			0/1			0/0		
Department Chairman	6			5			3			2			0			0		
Division Chief	6			8			16			14			0			0		
Academic Positions																		
Distinguished Professor	3			4			13			9			1			0		
Professor	7			20			31			30			4			0		
Associate Professor	1			4			10			23			33			1		
Assistant Professor	0			7			13			28			29			29		

Table 1

As in the prior Tables, the columns indicate specific time periods.

Graduates:

This row lists the total number of graduates for each period.

Academic Career:

The first row, initial, lists the number of graduates that chose to begin an academic career. The first entry is the total number followed by the percentage (initial/total). The data in parenthesis indicate the total number and the percent who began their career at Duke.

The second row, predominant, lists the number whose predominant career was academic and is followed by the percentage (predominant/initial). Data in parenthesis show the total number and percentage whose predominant career was at Duke.

Administrative Positions:

The next three rows list the administrative positions. The first row lists the number of Deans or Associate Deans; the second, Chairmen of Departments; the third, Division Chiefs. Note that an individual may be listed more than once, i.e., both a Division Chief and Chairman of a Department.

Academic Positions:

The next four rows list the highest academic rank. Note that only one entry per individual is possible for the ranks of Assistant Professor, Associate Professor or Professor. The Distinguished Professors are also included in the Professor designation.

Table 2 Career Choices in Fellow Subgroups (1946–2009)

Group	Number	Initial Academic Career	Predominant Academic Career
Total	564	58%	69%
Chief Medical Residents	95	65%	66%
Duke House Staff	194	58%	63%
Foreign	65	77%	84%
Clinical Research	270	67%	75%
Basic Research	161	73%	65%

Column 1 lists the total and subgroups analyzed.

Column 2 contains the total number of fellows in each subgroup.

Column 3 lists the % (initial/total) in each subgroup choosing an initial academic career.

Column 4 gives the % (predominant/initial) in each subgroup whose predominant career was spent in academia.

Table 3 Career Summary—Non-Academic

	1946–49	1960–69	1970–79	1980–89	1990–99	2000–09
Graduates (Total)	30	66	109	144	141	74
Non-Academic Careers						
Total	20 67%	40 60%	71 65%	85 59%	82 58%	32 43%
Practice	19	40	66	83	77	28
Other	1	0	5	2	5	4
Type of Practice						
Solo	12%	17%	12%	6%	8%	0%
Group	88%	83%	88%	94%	92%	100%
Former Duke Trainees in Group	29%	42%	40%	54%	54%	25%
Individual Practice						
General Cardiology	86%	86%	84%	50%	40%	39%
Primary Interventional	14%	5%	5%	31%	31%	43%
Primary Electrophysiology	0%	9%	11%	19%	29%	18%
Participation in Clinical Trials	22%	48%	73%	84%	85%	64%
Administrative Functions for Hospital	75%	74%	83%	78%	23%	7%
Administrative Functions for Practice	43%	42%	69%	54%	33%	0%
Participation in Professional Societies						
American College of Cardiology	67%	83%	93%	88%	92%	82%
Administrative Position in AHA or ACC	17%	11%	11%	14%	4%	0%
Clinical Appointments	6	13	47	44	12	6

Table 3

As in the prior tables, the columns indicate specific time periods.

Graduates:

This row lists the total number of graduates for each training period.

Non-Academic Careers:

The first row lists the total number of fellows and the percentage who pursued a predominately non-academic career.

The second and third rows list the number in practice and in other non-academic endeavors, respectively.

Type of Practice:

The percent in Solo (Row 1) or Group (Row 2) practice is listed, respectively.

The third row lists the percent of group practices with other Duke cardiology fellows.

Individual Practice:

General cardiology (may include diagnostic catheterization), primary interventional and primary electrophysiology are listed as a percent in the three rows, respectively.

Participation in Clinical Trials:

This row gives the percent participating in clinical trials.

Administrative Functions for the Hospital:

This row gives the percent having a significant administrative function as a hospital staff member such as Chief of Cardiology, Chief of Medicine, etc.

Administrative Functions for Practice:

This row lists the percent having a significant role in the administrative function of their practice.

Participation in Professional Societies:

Row 1 lists the percent who are Fellows of the American College of Cardiology. The second row lists the number having a significant role in the local or state American Heart Association or American College of Cardiology.

Clinical Appointments:

This row lists the percentage having a clinical appointment in an academic institution.

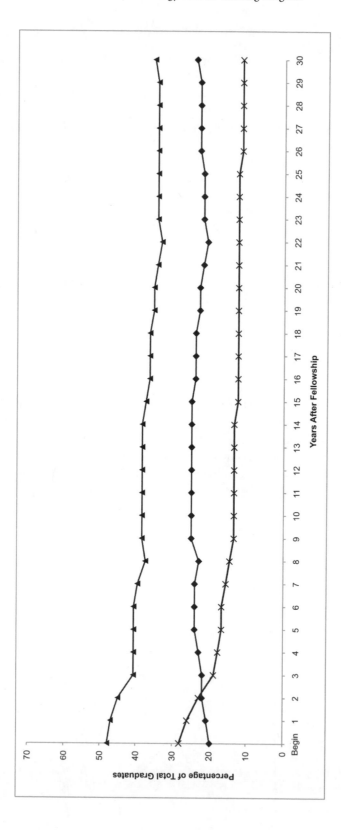

Figure 1 Thirty-year follow-up of the academic careers of 96 fellows finishing the Program between 1946–69. The percent in academic medicine (ordinate) each year during follow-up (abscissa) is depicted by the closed triangles, the percent at Duke by the Xs and the percent at other academic institutions by the closed diamonds.

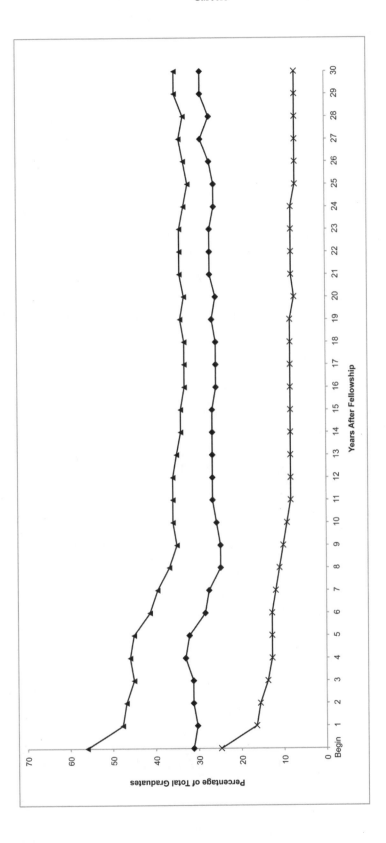

Figure 2 Thirty-year follow-up of the academic careers of 109 fellows finishing the Program between 1970–79. The format is the same as in Figure 1.

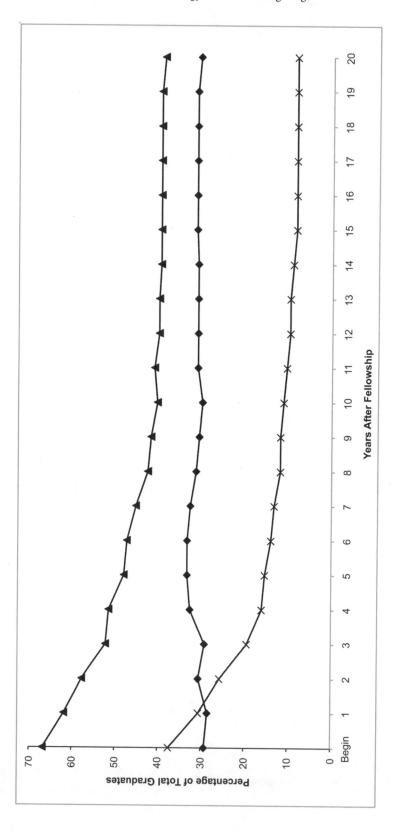

Figure 3 Twenty-year follow-up of the academic careers of 144 fellows finishing the Program between 1980–89. The format is the same as in Figure 1.

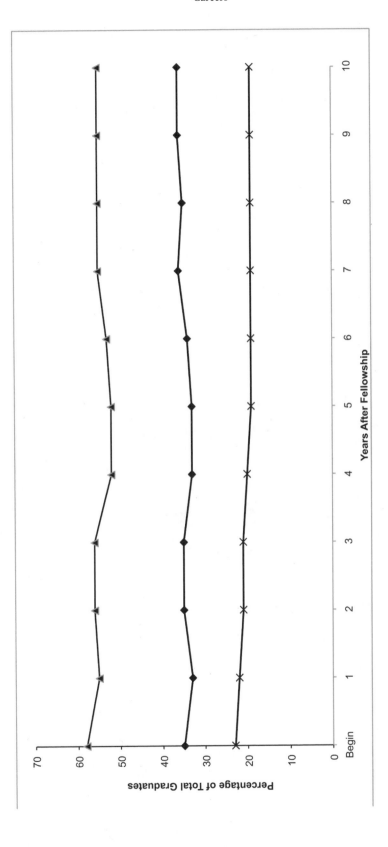

Figure 4 Ten-year follow-up of the careers of 141 fellows finishing the Program between 1990–99. The format is the same as in Figure 1.

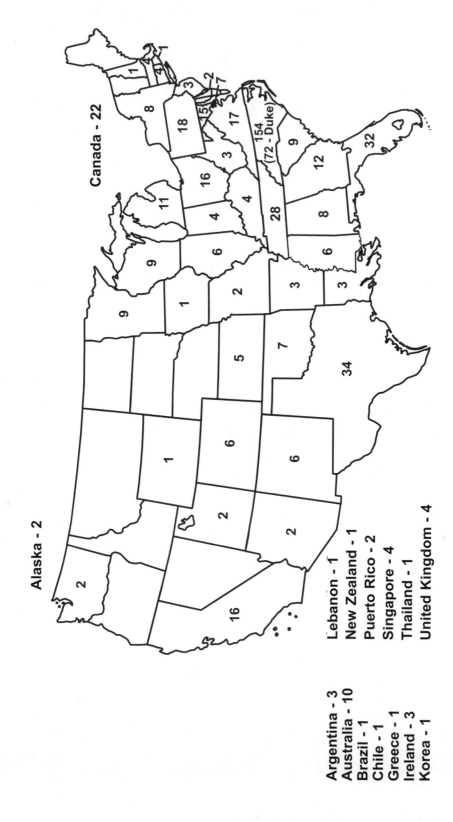

Figure 5 Figure 5 illustrates the geographic location of the predominant career of the former fellows who live within the United States. As might be anticipated, a large number, 154, settled in North Carolina and 72 spent their career at DUMC. At least one fellow was located in each of 39 states and in the District of Columbia. In addition, 55 fellows lived in 14 foreign countries, predominantly Canada and Australia.

CHAPTER XIV

PUBLICATIONS

The bibliography for each fellow was categorized as follows. Papers published during the period of the fellowship and for two years thereafter were considered work completed while a fellow. These papers were listed separately. Publications in which the fellows were either an author or co-author were counted and characterized as either peer review or not. No further characterization regarding specific scientific impact was attempted. Note that publications having more than one fellow as an author or co-author have been counted more than once.

In evaluating the bibliographies, only published research papers, editorials and book chapters were counted. No record of the number of abstracts was obtained. It should be noted that during their training, the fellows were encouraged to present at national meetings and many availed themselves of this opportunity. However, documenting the number of abstracts submitted and presentations made was not attempted.

The primary data on publications are listed in the Table and illustrated in the Figure. The percent of fellows publishing during their fellowship ranged from 85 to 97 and the number of papers published was quite similar during the six time periods. Those with specific research training and those who pursued a predominantly academic career were more productive regarding publications during their fellowship (Figure).

As would be expected, fellows who remained in academia published extensively during their career. Of interest is the large number of fellows pursuing a non-academic career who continued to publish scientific papers (range 30–87 percent for the time periods).

Publications

	1946–49	1960–69	1970–79	1980–89	1990–99	2000–09
Papers Published During Fellowship						
Percent Publishing	97	86	85	95	89	91
Mean (range)	4.6 (0–15)	4.3 (0–21)	5.8 (0–25)	8.2 (0–41)	8.1 (0–39)	6.9 (0–72)
Academic Career—Mean (range)	6.0 (2–9)	7.4 (1–21)	8.9 (0–20)	11 (0–41)	11.5 (0–39)	7.6 (0–48)
Non-Academic Career—Mean (range)	3.9 (0–15)	2.3 (0–10)	4.1 (0–25)	6.5 (0–22)	4.9 (0–20)	6.1 (0–72)
Papers Published During Career						
Academic						
Mean (range)	107 (24–237)	157 (1–787)	142 (16–590)	163 (5–1450)	57 (0–505)	18 (2–86)
Peer Reviewed (percent)	74	78	76	66	81	76
Non-Academic						
Mean (range)	16 (12–29)	13 (1–38)	23 (0–419)	23 (0–206)	9 (0–35)	11 (0–170)
Peer Reviewed (percent)	81	91	70	88	65	85
Continued to Publish (percent)	30	56	71	87	67	64

Table

Data are listed for each of the time periods as on the previous Tables.

The first category lists papers published during the fellowship and for a two-year period thereafter (mean and range). The percent of fellows publishing is listed in the first row. The mean number of papers and the range is given in the second row. The mean number of papers and the range for fellows with either an academic or a non-academic career are given in rows two and three, respectively.

The second category documents the number of papers published during their careers separated into predominantly academic and non-academic (mean and range). It should be noted that the number of career publications was somewhat skewed due to five individuals who affixed their name to a large number of papers.

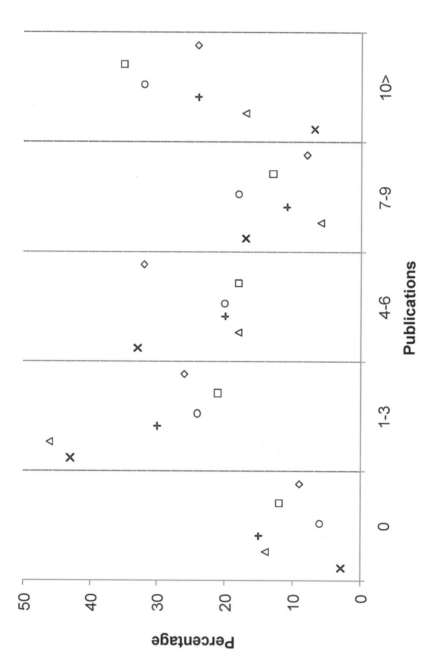

Figure The number of papers published during fellowship and for a two-year period thereafter, listed on the abscissa, are groups as follows: 0, 1–3, 4–6, 7–9, 10 and greater. The data are given as a percent of the total number of fellows training in a specific time period. The symbols denote the time period as follows: Xs 1946–59, Triangles 1960–69, Crosses 1970–79, Circles 1980–89, Squares 1990–99, and Diamonds 2000–09.

CHAPTER XV

CARDIOLOGY FELLOWS SOCIETY AND DUCCS

During the initial years of the Training Program, the majority of academic physicians attended the annual research meeting held at Atlantic City under the auspices of the "Young and Old Turks". However, this meeting was only sporadically attended by practicing physicians. The annual meeting of the American Heart Association (AHA), and later the American College of Cardiology, began to supplant the Atlantic City gatherings. By the early 1970s, these meetings were frequently attended by both practicing and academic cardiologists. Although theoretically the purpose of these meetings was for scientific interchange, the opportunity to visit with former colleagues became a major reason for attendance. As a consequence, informal gatherings of current and former Duke Fellows and faculty took place in one of the attendee's hotel rooms. The general format was to pick an evening, go to the local convenience store and buy potato chips, pretzels and beer. As the numbers increased, this approach became impractical; a larger meeting area was needed.

For several years the AHA meetings were held in Miami. The Division was able to use a yacht belonging a brother of Dr. Donald Hackel, a cardiac pathologist at Duke. One year a crisis occurred. The expected boat was at sea. Drs. Galen Wagner and Stan Anderson, an Australian cardiologist who was a frequent visitor to Duke, located a storage room in the Holiday Inn. Although the room was musty and filled with junk, they opened the doors and windows, put the junk on the balcony and a party site was unveiled. No fixtures, no furniture—nothing except a room in which the rug had a large hole in the middle. After covering the hole with a potted plant, found in the hall, and commandeering some furniture from several of their own rooms, the storage room became acceptable for the festivities. Tepid beer, wine, and a variety of junk foods were bought. The resulting party was judged as one of the best ever!

This semi-annual harum-scarum approach was finally solved by reserving a meeting room in which the hotel provided the refreshments. The logistical problems were solved; well-attended parties resulted. One serious problem remained: how to pay for the festivities?

In discussing solutions to this dilemma, a plan surfaced: develop a society of the former fellows in which annual dues would be used to support the cost of the two parties. The fellows were contacted and, in general, they supported this notion. Thus, in 1982 the Cardiology Fellows Society became a reality. In order to be certain that both the time and location of the party was known, a newsletter was sent to each of the members of the Fellows Society. The content of the newsletter, in addition to containing information regarding the parties, provided data about the fellows, both the incoming and those finishing the Program. One issue contained a key editorial ("More Than Twice a Year Cocktails") by Dr. Barry Ramo, which asked whether the Fellows Society should have additional functions beside party attendance. This editorial initiated a series of discussions. Finally, a group of former fellows was commissioned to discuss the issue and to formulate suggestions. The general consensus of this group: The Fellows Society should take on two academic missions: 1) provide postgraduate education for the fellows and 2) develop an opportunity for collaborative research.

In order to provide a format for continuing education, the Orgain Symposium began in 1982. This program evolved into a yearly gathering held on campus and chaired by Dr. Orgain as long as he was physically able. The format included an invited lecturer presented by one of the former fellows. A wide variety of topics were covered. The initial presentation made by Dr. Doug Zipes, outlined a history of the Training Program up to that juncture. Other presentations were given, usually by current members of the Duke faculty. Updates of current concepts of specific topics were given under the general rubric of "What's New in e.g., Electrophysiology". This Symposium was extremely well attended and continued for approximately ten years.

Several concurrent situations interacted so that the second objective, fostering collaborative research, became a reality. For several years, Dr. Stead had vociferously expressed his opinion that considerable money could be made by carrying out trials for the pharmaceutical industry. Dr. Malcolm Tyor, Chief of the Division of Gastroenterology, acted on this concept and developed a small consortium of his former fellows. They had worked with Clinical Research International, in the Research Triangle, to participate in a trial of Lovastatin. Additional trial sites were needed. Under the direction of Dr. David Pryor, who at that time had an administrative role in the Databank, and Galen, 24 former fellows, currently in practice, were recruited as test participants. This EXCEL trial was successfully completed and the general format for future trials established.

A group of the fellows expressed interest in fostering clinical research through the medium of trials. The Duke University Cooperative Cardiovascular Society (DUCCS) became a reality. The organization elected a President and board of Directors. Membership required either a significant initial financial contribution or functioning as principal investigator in one of the clinical trials. In addition, several of the Duke faculty participated in various administrative roles. The DUCCS organization was responsible for allocating expenditure of surplus funds from the trials. The Division of Cardiology's primary role was to deal with the pharmaceutical industry, to initiate the trials and to act as coordinator. Dr. Chris O'Connor was designated as the primary coordinator of the trials. A newsletter describing the DUCCS activities was published by Galen for several years.

The DUCCS organization continued to expand, so that by 1988, 146 of the former trainees became members. Membership in DUCCS was expanded to include former Duke faculty, a number of regional physicians who referred patients to Cardiology at Duke and colleagues of DUCCS members. For several years, money was available to support a cardiology fellow.

A number of clinical trials were carried out to evaluate modalities employed for either the diagnosis or therapy of cardiovascular disease. The Table lists the acronyms for these trials and the number of former fellows participating as site principal investigators in each trial. This list includes only those trials in which DUCCS played a major role, providing either all of the study sites or an extensive network within a larger group of sites.

A second component of the DUCCS activities included a variety of investigator initiated clinical research projects. Perhaps the most notable was carried out by Dr. Staff Warren, who measured the effects on the electrocardiogram due to prolonged occlusion of a coronary artery by balloon inflation. A number of publications and two PhD candidates finished their research work from the data obtained in "The Staff Studies".

An additional project to define the genetics of cardiovascular disease was instituted by Dr. Bill Kraus under the rubric of GENECARD. A number of the DUCCS investigators have provided patient material to be incorporated into this database.

During the latter part of the 90s, interest in the educational aspects of the Cardiology Fellows Society waned. The Orgain Symposium, which had been discontinued, was resurrected under the rubric of the Wallace Symposium. This meeting, primarily related to issues of cardiac rehabilitation, was held yearly from 2000 to 2005. Other educational activities were not continued. By 2006, the Cardiology Fellows Society essentially disappeared as a functioning entity and was incorporated into DUCCS. The annual gatherings at the national Cardiology meetings were supported by either the Division or the DCRI.

During the initial five years of this century, DUCCS continued to be a functioning unit, although somewhat reduced in scope. Drs. Steve Roark and Alan Chu provided external leadership and were successful in raising a significant amount of money through sites involved in clinical trials. A number of former fellows continued to work directly with the DCRI and did not go though the DUCCS organization. For a three year period, 2005–2008, DUCCS had no formal external leadership but was kept functional through the efforts of Galen.

In 2008, DUCCS went through another reorganization. Drs. John Heitner, Ricky Schneider and Sebastian Palmeri became President, Vice President and Treasurer, respectively. Drs. Doug Schocken and George Adams were appointed to provide liaison to the faculty of the Cardiology Division. The new leadership initiated a return to a membership fee. Currently, there are 271 active members of DUCCS; 70 percent had been Duke Cardiology Fellows. The membership of DUCCS has also been subdivided into specific areas of interest. Currently there are four subgroups: DAVINCI—imaging, StentaDUCCS—intervention, ElectroDUCCS—electrophysiology, and Mal-HEARTS—heart failure. Several new clinical studies have been initiated, bringing the total to 12 active trials. (Table) At this writing, the organization appears to be on another ascending limb of activity.

The continued success of DUCCS is unique to the Cardiology Division at Duke. A number of other academic training programs have tried to develop similar approaches with their fellows, but to date, the results have been only marginally successful.

DUCCS Trials

Name of Trial	# Fellows
APSAC	13
CARS	30
PRAISE I	36
APSAC II	8
PAC TACH	17
IMPACT II	28
EXCEL	24
PRIME	11
LEXUS	11
AFIB	7
SAD HEART	7
PURSUIT	35
ENTICES	6
PRAISE II	37
DOFETILIDE 128	8
ATLAST	16
HARE	6
RENAAL	6
GENECARD*	11
OPTIME*	12
ACTIV*	4
RITZ4*	8
ST-MAP*	15
TIME-MC*	7
RELY*	49
TOPCAT*	25
RELY-ABLE*	26
SMART-3*	2
TTR*	10
HYPERCISE*	7

The acronym describing the specific trial is listed along with the number of fellows participating in the trial. An asterisk indicates that the trial is active.

CHAPTER XVI

CARDIOLOGY RESEARCH FELLOWS

Throughout the period encompassed by this study, there were a large number of separate research laboratories, both clinical and basic. As noted previously, the majority of cardiology trainees obtained specific research training in these venues during their fellowship. In addition, there were a number of cardiologists who received <u>only</u> research training in one or more of these laboratories. Table 1 gives descriptive data on 57 of these individuals. Of the 55 who finished their research training, 84 percent currently are pursuing an academic career.

The research laboratories in the Cardiology Division were active in training a large number of medical students. In addition, a number of candidates received their PhD degree or had a post-doctoral fellowship in cardiology laboratories. A list of these individuals is beyond the scope of this work. However, it should be noted that many of them made a major impact on both the research productivity of these laboratories and were intimately involved in training the cardiology fellows to carry out meaningful research.

Table 1 Cardiology Research Fellows

Name	Institution	Fellowship Dates	Mentor	Research	Initial Career	Subsequent Career
Attramadal, Havard	Rikshospitalet University Hosp., Oslo, Norway	1990–93*	Lefkowitz	B	A	A
Baeza, Ricardo G.	Catholic University, Santiago, Chile	2003–06*	Krucoff	C	A	A
Barbagelata, Alejandro	Hospital Italiano, Buenos Aires, Argentina	1993–94*	Califf	C	P	P
Bates, Michael P.	Monogram Biosciences Inc. San Francisco	1992–94	Stiles	B	O	OMI
Benjamin, Ivor J.	U. Utah School of Medicine Salt Lake City	1988–90*	Willliams	B	A	A
Brown, James E.	U. Western Ontario, Canada	1980–82*	Shand	B	A	A
Chauhan, Vijay S.	Toronto General Hosp., Ontario, Canada	1997–99*	Grant	B	A	A
Cho, Myeong-Chen	Chungbuk National University, Korea	1996–98*	Rockman	B	A	A
Choi, Dong-Ju	Chungbuk National University, Korea	1995–98*	Rockman	B	A	A
Clemmensen, Peter	U. Copenhagen, Denmark	1992–94*	Wagner	C	A	A
Corvoisier, Philippe Le	INSERM Unit 400, Creteil, France	2001–03*	Rockman	B	A	A
Curcio, Antonio	Catanzaro, Italy	2004–05*	Rockman	B	A	A
Deb, Arjun	U. North Carolina	2005–07*	Dzau	B	A	A
dos Santos, Fabio Cesar	Hospital Unicor., Sao Paulo, Brazil	1998–99*	Ryan	B	A	A
Engblom, Henrik	U. Lund, Sweden	2004–06*	Wagner	C	A	A
Esposito, Giovanni	Federico II U. Naples, Italy	1998–00*	Rockman	B	A	A

Name	Institution	Fellowship Dates	Mentor	Research	Initial Career	Subsequent Career
Feldman, David S.	Cardiology Division The Ohio State University	1999–01*	Lefkowitz/Rockman	B	A	A
Firek, Bohdan M.	Academy of Medicine, Warsaw, Poland	1996–97*	Kisslo	C	A	A
Grande, Peer	U. Copenhagen, Denmark	1980–82*	Wagner	C	A	A
Guadalajra, Jose F. •	Mexico	1979–80*	Kisslo	C	A	A
Hakacova, Nina	Comenius University, Slovakia	2008–09*	Wagner	C	A	A
Helmy, Sherif	Cairo Universtiy, Egypt	1986–87*	Kisslo	C	P	P
Holmvang, Lene	U. Copenhagen, Denmark	1998–00*	Wagner	C	A	A
Iaccarino, Guido	Federico II U. Naples, Italy	1996–99*	Lefkowitz	B	A	A
Ismail, Suad A.	Subbiah Cardiology Assoc., Butler, PA	1990–92*	Kisslo	C	P	P
Johanson, Per	Sahlgrenska University, Sweden	2001–03*	Krucoff	C	A	A
Jurlander, Birgit	U. Copenhagen, Denmark	1996–98*	Wagner	C	OMI	A
Kang, Duk Hyun	Seoul National University, Korea	1999–00*	Ryan	C	A	A
Kavanaugh, Katherine M.	U. Alberta, Edmonton, Alberta, Canada	1988–90*	Ideker	B	A	A
Kim, Han Woong	Northwestern Memorial Hosp.	2005–06*	Kim	C	A	A
Klicpera, Martin	U. Vienna, Austria	1977–78*	Kisslo	C	A	A
Kuijt, Wichert J.	Academic Medical Center Amsterdam, The Netherlands	2008–p*	Krucoff	C		
Lebeau, Real	U. Montreal, Canada	1979–80*	Kisslo	C	A	A
Lotfi, Hekmat	U. Toronto, Canada	2002–04*	Jollis	C	A	A
Majidi, Mohamed	Maastricht University, The Netherlands	2005–08	Krucoff	C	O	O

Name	Institution	Fellowship Dates	Mentor	Research	Initial Career	Subsequent Career
Matsushita, Kenichi	Keio University School of Medicine Tokyo, Japan	2004–07*	Dzau	B	A	A
Martin, Thomas	U. Glasgow, Scotland	2007–09*	Wagner	C	A	A
Melloni, Chiara	Duke Medical Center	2005–07*	Harrington	C	A	A
Noma, Takashisa	Kagawa University, Japan	2003–06*	Rockman	B	A	A
Ohta, Takahiro	Tokyo Medical University, Japan	1992–98*	Ryan	C	P	P
Oliveira, Gustavo Bernardes de Figueiredo	Federal University of Uberlandia, Brazil	2002–05*	Granger	C	A	A
Park, Hyun-Young	Yonsei Cardiovascular Research Institute, Korea	2002–03*	Rockman	B	A	A
Perrino, Cinzia	Federico II U. Naples, Italy	2002–05*	Rockman	B	A	A
Persson, Eva	U. Lund, Sweden	2002–04*	Wagner	C	A	A
Pettersson, Jonas	U. Lund, Sweden	1997–99*	Wagner	C	A	OMI
Rapacciuolo, Antonio	Federico II U. Naples, Italy	1997–00*	Rockman	B	A	A
Roussakis, George •	U. Athens, Greece	1997–98*	Ryan	C		
Sadick, Norman	Blacktown Hosp., New South Wales, Australia	1982–85*	Greenfield	B	P	P
Saint-Jacques, Henock	Mount Sinai, NYC	2001–03*	Harrington	C	A	A
Sogade, Felix O.	Macon, GA	1995–96*	Grant	B	P	P
Strasser, Ruth H.	U. Dresden, Germany	1982–85*	Lefkowitz	B	A	A
Szwed, Hanna	Polish Institute of Cardiology, Poland	1986–87*	Kisslo	C	A	A
Takaoka, Hideyuki	Kobe University School of Medicine, Japan	1999–01*	Rockman	B	A	A

Name	Institution	Fellowship Dates	Mentor	Research	Initial Career	Subsequent Career
Tragardh, Elin	U. Lund, Sweden	2003–05*	Wagner	C	A	A
Tricoci, Pierluigi	U. Bologna, Italy	2004–06*	Harrington	C	A	A
Weinstaft, Jonathan W.	Weill Cornell Medical Center	2003–04*	Kim	C	A	A
White, James A.	London Health Sciences Center London, Ontario, Canada	2005–07*	Kim	C	A	A

See "Explanation for Data Tables" following Chapter II. The Institution column gives the current location of the individual rather than the location of prior clinical training.

APPENDIX

SOURCES

The purpose of this section is to document the extensive source material utilized in this book. Data will be given as either general or specific to a given chapter.

Before proceeding, a caveat is in order. Although every effort was made to obtain complete and validated data, undoubtedly, the results are not perfect. If any individual is either missing or miscast, an apology is in order.

General

The first task was to obtain a complete list of the trainees. In compiling these data, with two exceptions, the trainees were included if they participated in the Training Program for at least a year. The trainees are listed for a specific time period in the Tables associated with Chapters II–VII and Chapter XVI. Multiple, but incomplete, lists were obtained from a variety of sources and were carefully collated. The most extensive and correct data were provided by Paul Thacker and Sandra Mangum of the Department of Medicine (based on the funding of the trainees). In fact, without these data, our job would have been essentially impossible.

Additional lists were provided by Drs. Galen Wagner, Joe Kisslo, Tom Ryan, Bob Lefkowitz, Marcus Wharton, Kevin Harrison, Tom Bashore and Howard Rockman.

A website (cardiofellows@mc.duke.edu), which gives personal data on a number of the fellows, has been developed by Dr. Tom Bashore. (The material obtained from our research has been used to update this database.)

A very important source was the fellow training assignments 1968 to present. These data were utilized to cross-check the dates of participation by the fellows and to denote the curriculum for a given individual.

Current demographic information was obtained from a variety of sources. When possible, each fellow was contacted to verify pertinent facts regarding their training (approximately 95% contacted). In addition, a current curriculum vitae and bibliography was obtained on the majority.

The Directory of the American Board of Medical Specialists and the North Carolina Medical Board databases were extremely helpful.

Several individuals in the Medical Media Section of the Durham Veterans Affairs Medical Center provided outstanding support. Access to medical databases and invaluable assistance extracting data was provided by Jeffrey Kager, Chief Library Service and Stephen Perlman, Librarian. In addition, Lesa Hall, the medical illustrator, formatted the illustrations and photographs.

Other sources include: The Duke Medical Alumni Office, Who's Who in America, membership lists of the American Society for Clinical Investigation, American Physiological Society, American College of Cardiology, Council on Clinical Cardiology of the American Heart Association.

During the period February 2002–June 2009, I recorded a detailed interview with a number of fellows and faculty either directly or via telephone. Their insight regarding the fellowship was extraordinarily helpful in formulating the text.

The following individuals were contacted:

Thomas M. Bashore	Christopher M. O'Connor
Victor S. Behar	Robert H. Peter
Michael A. Blazing	Edward L.C. Pritchett
Christopher H. Cabell	David B. Pryor
Robert M. Califf	William W. Pryor
A. Alan Chu	Barry W. Ramo
Mark P. Donahue	Robert A. Rosati
E. Harvey Estes	Michael Rotman
Walter L. Floyd	Thomas Ryan
Marcel R. Gilbert	Douglas D. Schocken
Pascal Goldschmidt	C. Frank Starmer
Augustus O. Grant	Eugene A. Stead
Stephen C. Hammill	Gary L. Stiles
James G. Jollis	Howard K. Thompson
Joseph A. Kisslo	Galen S. Wagner
William E. Kraus	Andrew G. Wallace
Kerry L. Lee	John M. Wallace
Daniel B. Mark	Andrew Wang
Henry D. McIntosh	Robert A. Waugh
Julie M. Miller	Menashe B. Waxman
James J. Morris	Arnold M. Weissler
Kenneth G. Morris	K. Michael Zabel

Specific to a Chapter

Chapter I

1. Gifford, Jr., James F.: *The Evolution of a Medical Center. The History of Medicine at Duke University to 1941.* Duke University Press. Durham, North Carolina 1972.

2. Synopsis of Edward Orgain's Contributions to Duke Medical Center (written for the institution of the Edward S. Orgain Distinguished Professorship).

Chapter II

1. Pryor, William W.: My Recollections of Being an Orgain Fellow in Cardiovascular Disease 1953–55 (written July 1999).

Chapter VII

Procedure volume was provided by Dr. Jimmy Tcheng.

Chapter X

Training Grant HL007101-35. Unfortunately, only a paragraph summary of the initial training grants (HEO5736 and HEO5369) are available.

Data regarding NIH research and training grants were obtained through the CRISP (Computer Retrieval of Information on Scientific Projects) (commons.cit.nih.gov./crisp3) database maintained by the office of Extramural Research at the National Institute of Health. This database contains a listing of NIH grants from 1972–present. Grants obtained prior to that time are listed only if the recipient was at Duke and "word of mouth" information was available.

Linda Wilkins and Ellen Brearley were instrumental in obtaining the NIH grant information.

Comprehensive data regarding the funding of cardiology fellows by the American Heart Association were provided by Marsha Baker and Ellen Brearley. Note that grants of cardiology fellows at other academic institutions have not been included.

An estimate of the research support of the fellows from the Veterans Affairs Medical Center was obtained from the Research and Development Service and through review of the curriculum vitae of the fellows.

Chapter XI

Source material and demographic map were provided by Susan Lee Greenfield.

Chapter XII

Data regarding the requirements for certification in Cardiovascular Disease by the American Board of Internal Medicine were provided by Elizabeth Hopkins, Associate Vice President, and Dr. Harry R. Kimball, President of the American Board of Internal Medicine.

Board certifications were obtained via the American Board of Internal Medicine website, ABIM.org.

Chapter XIII

1. Pritchett, Edward L.C., Galen S. Wagner, Andrew G. Wallace and Joseph C. Greenfield, Jr.: Career Choices of 135 Cardiology Trainees at Duke University Medical Center from 1970–1984. Am J. Cardiol 57(No. 4):313–315, February 1986.

The following survey was sent to a number the majority of the fellows who are currently in practice. Question 8. also was sent to a number of fellows in academic medicine. A total of 358 surveys were sent and 72 percent were completed and returned.

1. Type of practice:
   - ☐ Solo
   - ☐ Group

   If group:
   - ☐ Limited to Cardiology
   - ☐ Multispecialty

2. Other Duke Cardiology fellows in group:
   ☐ Yes
   ☐ No

3. Your practice:
   ☐ General cardiology – no invasive procedures
   ☐ General cardiology with invasive procedures
   ☐ Primarily intervention
   ☐ Primarily electrophysiology

4. Research:

   Have you participated in:
   ☐ DUCCS research project
   ☐ Other clinical trials

5. Role in administrative functions for your hospital:
   ☐ Chief of Cardiology
   ☐ Chief of Medicine
   ☐ Member of IRB Committee
   ☐ Member of Ethics Committee
   ☐ Other (please specify)

6. Role in administrative functions for your practice group:
   ☐ Chief of Cardiology
   ☐ Other (please specify)

7. Participation in professional societies:
   ☐ American Heart Association
   ☐ Local or statewide officer in American Heart Association
   ☐ Member of the American College of Cardiology
   ☐ Local or statewide officer in American College of Cardiology
   ☐ Other (Please list.)

8. We are interested in defining factors which may have affected your career choice, academic vs. practice.

   Debt at the beginning of cardiology fellowship (corrected to the 1980 dollar value)
   ☐ Less than $25,000
   ☐ $25,000–$50,000
   ☐ Greater than $50,000

   Were you married at the beginning of your cardiology fellowship?
   ☐ Yes
   ☐ No

   Had you made a definite decision regarding practice or academic at the beginning of the fellowship?
   ☐ Yes
   ☐ No

   If not, were you leaning toward academic vs. practice?
   ☐ Yes
   ☐ No

Had you had basic research experience?

- ☐ None
- ☐ Undergraduate
- ☐ Medical school
- ☐ House staff training

Had you had clinical research experience?

- ☐ None
- ☐ Undergraduate
- ☐ Medical school
- ☐ House staff training

Chapter XIV

The databases of the Library of Medicine (ncbi/nlm.nih.gov) and google.com were utilized to obtain a list of each fellow's publications. Individual bibliographies were obtained from a majority of the fellows and used as cross-references. In addition, the bibliographies of Drs. Orgain, McIntosh, Estes and Greenfield were used to obtain publications by the fellows during training.

Chapter XV

A list of the fellows who participated in DUCCS Trials was obtained through Galen Wagner and Kathy Shuping.

"Rogues' Gallery"

A number of photographs of fellows and faculty were taken at various social functions primarily by Dr. Bob Waugh. The pictures of faculty engaged in hospital activities were obtained from a number of individuals.

"Rogues' Gallery"

The following contains photographs of fellows (137) and faculty responsible for the Training Program, either at work or play—mostly play. The percent of fellows pictured for each decade ranges from 14 to 30.

The decade in which the picture was taken is identified by a number on each caption as follows: 1 (1946–59), 2 (1960–69), 3 (1970–79), 4 (1980–89), 5 (1990–1999), 6 (2000–2009). An asterisk denotes individuals who were not members of the fellowship.

The choice from a large collection was entirely random. Any fellows not shown should **not** conclude that they are too ugly to appear!

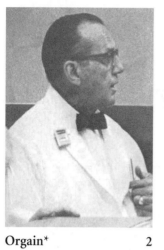

Orgain*   2

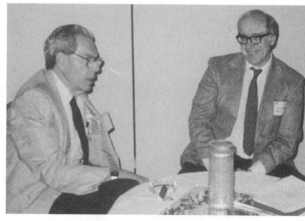

McIntosh   Wagner   5

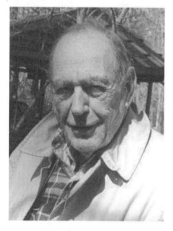

Stead*   5

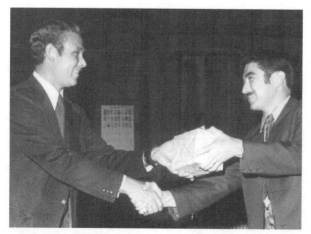

J. Gallagher   Schocken   McIntosh   4

A. Wallace   Simon   3

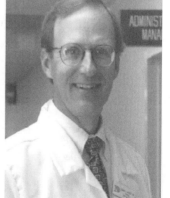

Pritchett   4

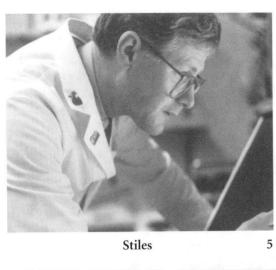

Stiles   5

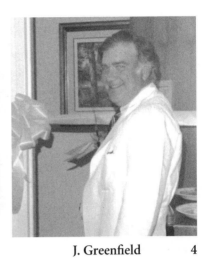

J. Greenfield   4

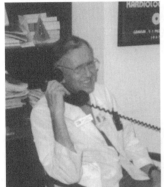

Peter   4

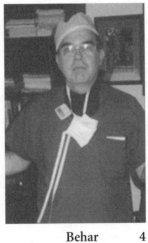

Behar   4

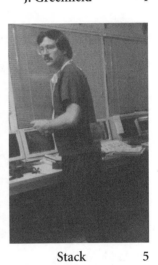

Stack   5

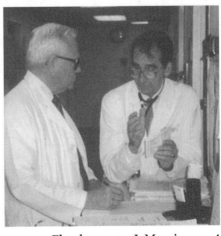

Bashore   Ohman   5

Floyd   J. Morris   4

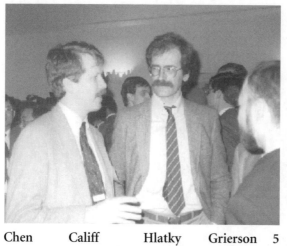

Chen   Califf   Hlatky   Grierson   5

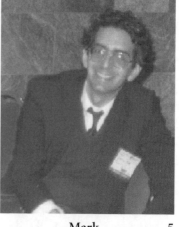

Mark   5

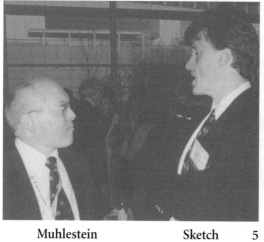

Muhlestein   Sketch   5

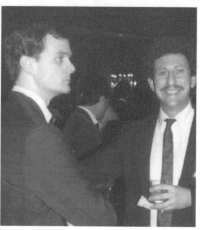

Packer   Sintetos   4

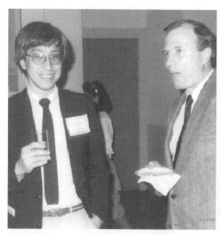

Chu   Lee*   4

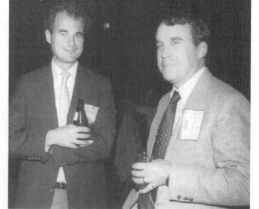

Parker   Seaworth   4

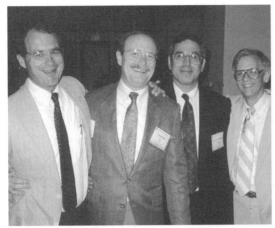

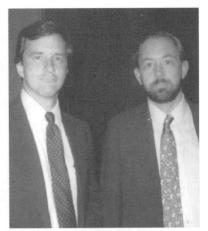

Parker   Wise   Prystowsky Fraker 4   Skelton   K. Morris   4

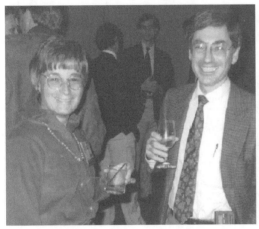
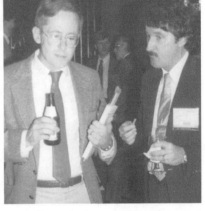

Swain   R. Davidson 4   Guarnieri   Bramlet   4

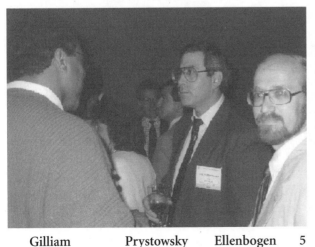
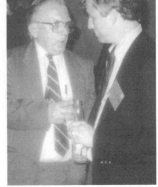

Gilliam   Prystowsky   Ellenbogen 5   S. Anderson* O'Connor 5

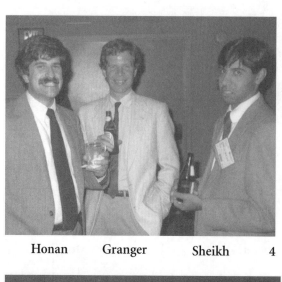

Honan   Granger   Sheikh   4

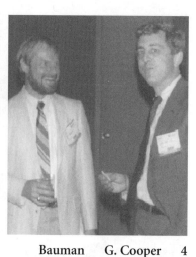

Bauman   G. Cooper   4

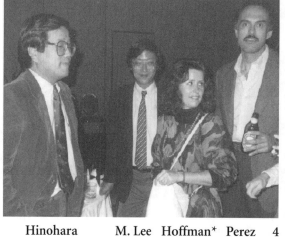

Hinohara   M. Lee Hoffman* Perez   4

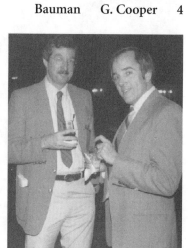

Cobb   Gibbons   4

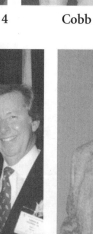
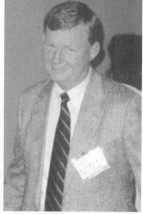

Lieppe   Dugan   Waugh   McGrew   4

Kendall   5

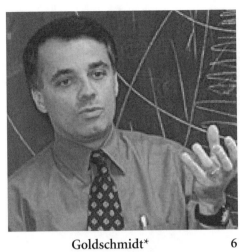

Goldschmidt* 6

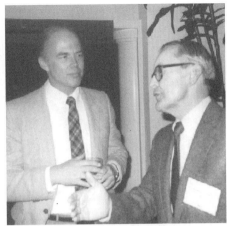

Hartman   Maha   4

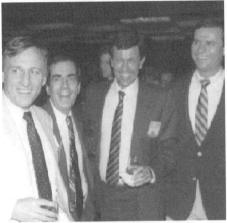

Bethea   Kisslo   Tonkin   Juk   4

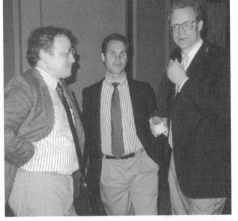

Fortin   Frid   Wall   5

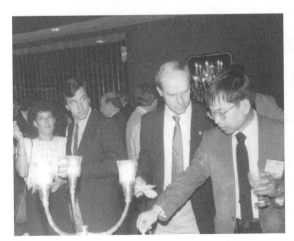

Hurwitz   Skelton   Parsons   Chen   4

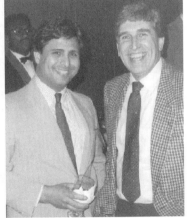

Vidaillet   M. Gilbert   4

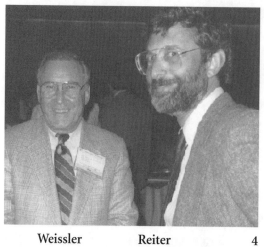

Weissler   Reiter   4

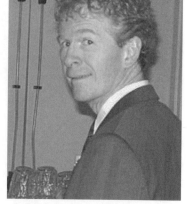

Ryan*   5

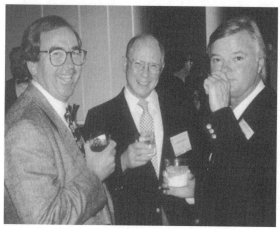

Bennett   Miller   B. Johnson   5

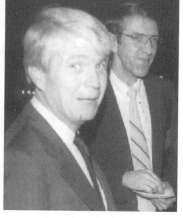

Dugan   Warren   4

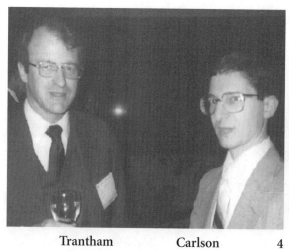

Trantham   Carlson   4

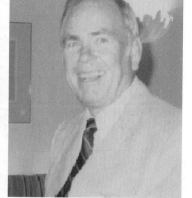

Sleeper   4

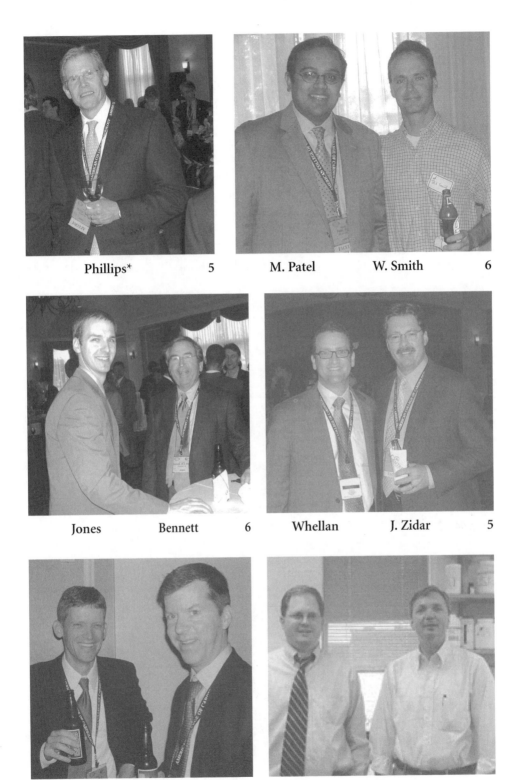

Phillips* 5

M. Patel W. Smith 6

Jones Bennett 6

Whellan J. Zidar 5

L. Allen Felker 6

Wolf Rockman* 6

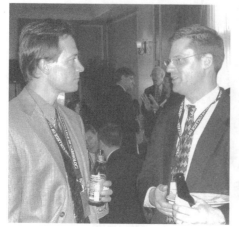

Povsic   G. Adams   6

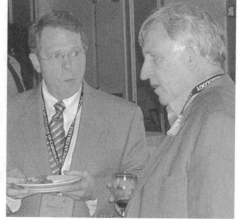

Bashore   Bethea   5

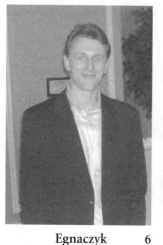

Egnaczyk   6

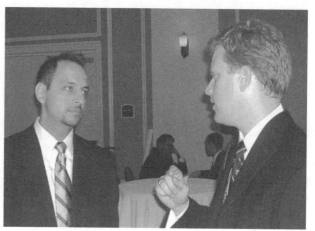

Kaul   Brennan   6

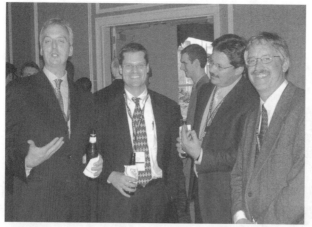

Kandzari   G. Adams   Jones   J. Zidar   W. Baker   6

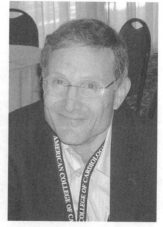

Sprecher   5

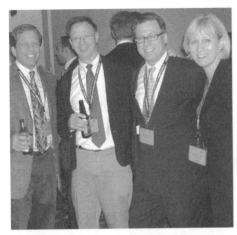

Lieberman Thel Negus* G. Peterson 5

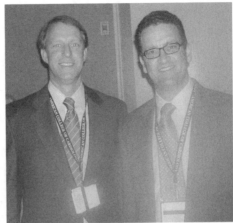

Markham   Whellan   5

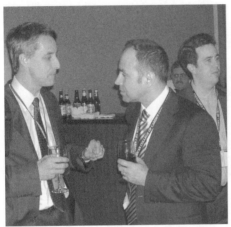

Mahaffey   Goodman* Hernandez 6

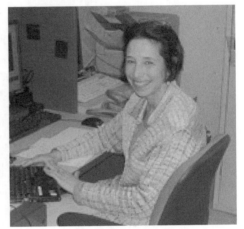

P. Douglas*   6

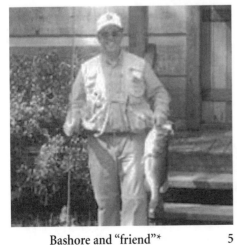

Bashore and "friend"*   5

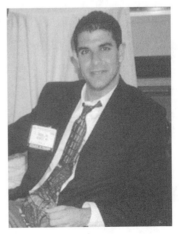

Rebeiz   6

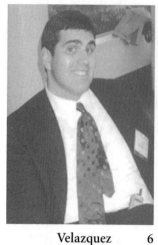

Velazquez   6

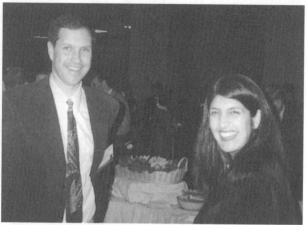

Krasuski   M. Shah   6

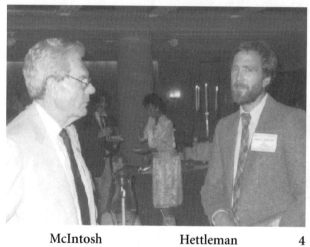

McIntosh   Hettleman   4

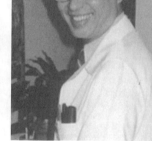

Kong   4

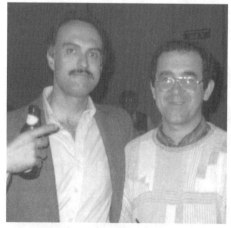

Perez   Quigley   4

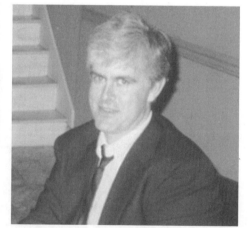

K. Harrison   4

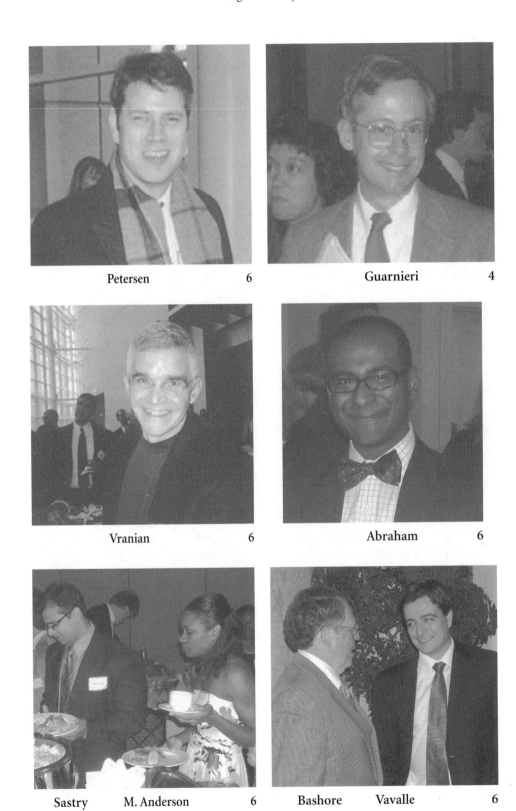

Petersen 6

Guarnieri 4

Vranian 6

Abraham 6

Sastry   M. Anderson   6

Bashore   Vavalle   6

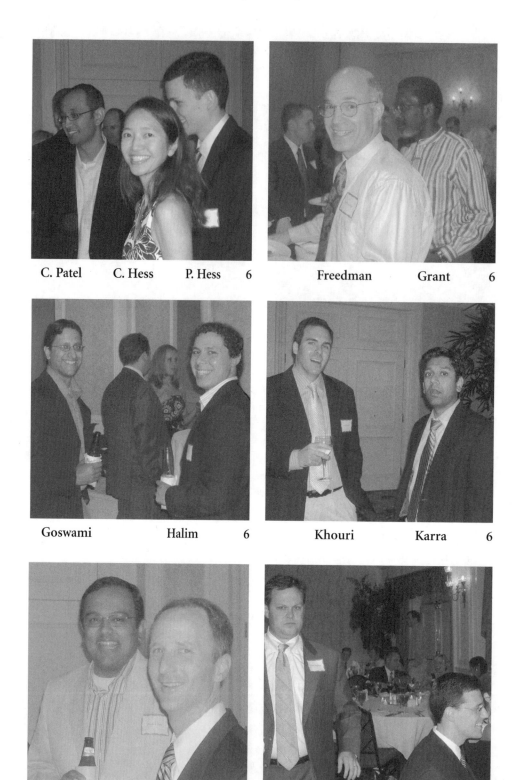

C. Patel C. Hess P. Hess 6

Freedman Grant 6

Goswami Halim 6

Khouri Karra 6

M. Patel Mills 6

Mulhearn Mudrick 6

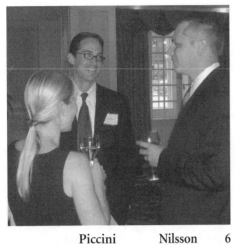

Piccini   Nilsson   6

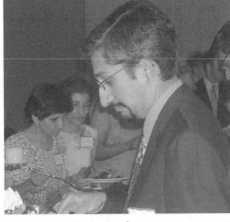

Rajagopal   6

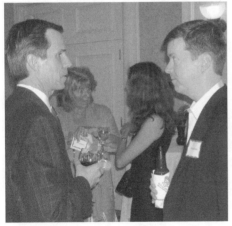

Rogers*   Felker   6

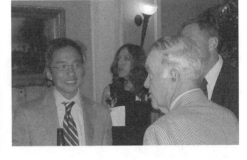

A. Wang   J. Greenfield   6

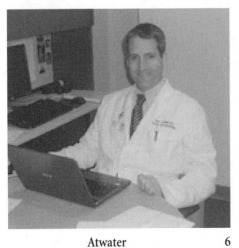

Atwater   6

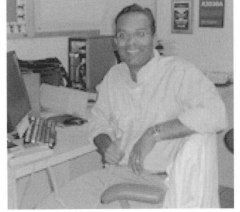

Rao   6

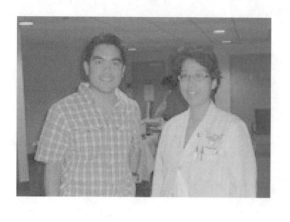 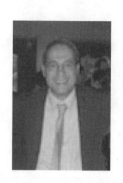

Sun   T. Wang   6   Stiber   6

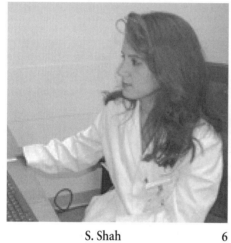 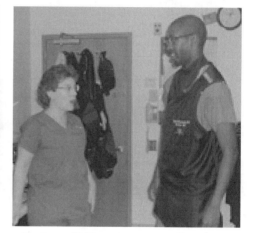

S. Shah   6   R. Greenfield   E. Williams   6

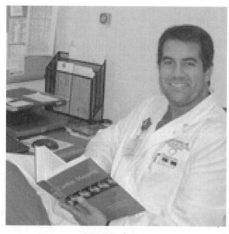 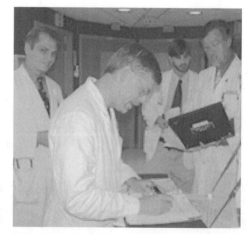

Hranitzky   6   Nilsson   Gehrig   Huff*   Blalock*   6

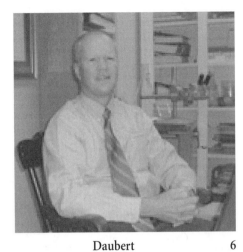

Daubert 6

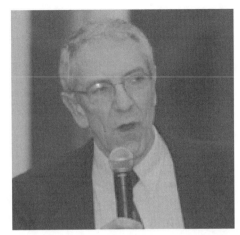

Warren 6

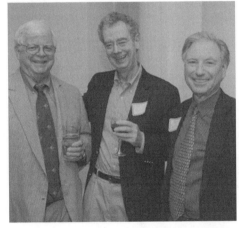

Waugh   Rosati   R. Davidson 6

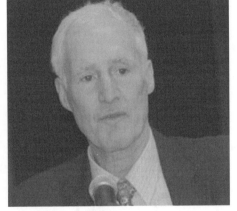

Brenner 6

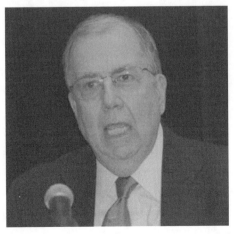

Kisslo 6

Epilogue

There is one very obvious conclusion that can be drawn from this material: the Duke Cardiology Fellows Training Program has produced an extraordinarily impressive and talented group of cardiologists. During the past sixty-three years, these physicians have made a major impact on the care of patients with cardiovascular disease, at DUMC and at many national and international locations. The fellows have amassed an impressive record in both academia and practice. Although comparative data are not available for similar training programs, it is doubtful if any could surpass this track record.

What are the responsible factors leading to this level of success? There is no simple answer. As with any endeavor of this type, two components are key: recruitment of the best people and the content of the Training Program—nature vs. nurture. Although both are important, it is essentially impossible from the data examined to determine which of these two is paramount. My own prejudice: it is the former.

The nature of cardiology has changed so dramatically during the duration of the Program that it is hardly recognizable. However, the training endeavors have not only kept pace with the changes, but have been responsible for moving the field in a positive direction.

The faculty at Duke has been drawn in large measure from the Training Program—72 graduates spent their predominant career at Duke. Obviously, the dedication of this faculty to the Training Program, serving as mentors and role models, has been a major force in producing these outstanding results. Many specific characteristics of the Training Program were examined, but a precise definition of the key factors leading to an academic choice was not forthcoming.

The credentials as an academic training program are unquestioned: approximately 40 percent of the graduates have pursued a predominant career in academia. Based on the prior record, I am confident that in the future, cardiology will be markedly influenced and well served by the graduates of the Duke Cardiology Fellows Training Program.